How to Facilitate Lifestyle Change

How to Facilitate Lifestyle Change

Applying Group Education in Healthcare

Amanda Avery, RD
Senior Fellow of the Higher Education Academy
Assistant Professor in Nutrition and Dietetics
Division of Nutritional Sciences
University of Nottingham
Loughborough, UK

Kirsten Whitehead, PhD, RD
Senior Fellow of the Higher Education Academy
Assistant Professor in Dietetics
School of Biosciences
Division of Nutritional Sciences
University of Nottingham
Loughborough, UK

Vanessa Halliday, PhD, RD
Senior Fellow of the Higher Education Academy
Lecturer in Public Health
School of Health and Related Research (ScHARR)
The University of Sheffield
Sheffield, UK

WILEY Blackwell

Contents

Chapter 8: Managing group interaction and how to overcome challenges, 150

Vanessa Halliday

Chapter 9: Personal development in group facilitation skills, 166

Amanda Avery

Foreword

Working and learning together within a small group is a less resource intensive and a more accessible and acceptable form of education for many individuals. Groups can be considered to be very much like teams where there are people taking part who have similar ambitions and needs, aiming to achieve similar goals.

The publication of this guide is timely, with the current highest emphasis on prevention and health improvement this century. The *Five Year Forward View*, published by Simon Stevens (Chief Executive of NHS England) last year, states that the future health of millions of children, the sustainability of the NHS, and the economic prosperity of Britain all now depend on a radical upgrade in prevention and public health. The World Health Organisation, the European Platform for Health and the USA Centers for Disease Control and prevention all also recognize that many of the non-communicable diseases, which are contributing to health and societal burden, are preventable or better managed through improved self-care. Chapter 1 provides startling global statistics of the need for lifestyle change to be championed and delivered at every opportunity through a range of scalable solutions using a life-course approach. The principles of behaviour change then set the scene for the reader to walk through the stages of group education with the three authors.

Today, the range of professionals delivering lifestyle advice is wider than ever before, as we embrace concepts such as Making Every Contact Count. The skills that lifestyle educators and health professionals require in order to deliver effective group education and support are clearly transferable from other interactions, such as one to one consultations, but require adaptation and a broader focus. This concise and highly practical resource guides the reader through each stage requiring consideration; from planning to delivery of a session with appropriate resources through to evaluation.

Groups have additional advantages over the traditional one-to-one approach in that the participants can become committed and motivated to help others. Facilitators can harness peer support and encourage the lay person, with training and support, to facilitate groups as a critical and effective strategy for lifestyle change, as well as ongoing health care and the benefits being cascaded at a local community level.

I trust that as you utilize this resource, you will be inspired and better informed about how to implement group education and that this additional competence will contribute to your ongoing personal development. The advice offered for overcoming challenging situations and the ambivalent group member, will be best reflected upon in practice!

Additionally, and most importantly, I hope that your group participants will benefit from your best practice and the motivating power and extra resolve developed through peer support facilitating sustained behaviour change. I celebrate the publication of this book with the authors, who are all outstanding dietetic practitioners, communicators and educators.

Dr Fiona McCullough
Director of Dietetics, The University of Nottingham
Principal Fellow of the Higher Education Academy
Chair of the British Dietetic Association

Preface

The prevention and management of non-communicable diseases, that are being seen across all societies and which result from poor lifestyle habits, requires scalable and effective solutions. Small changes, in the healthier direction, to improved dietary habits, increased physical activity levels, decreased sedentary behaviours, safer alcohol intake and a decreased number of people smoking may considerably reduce the prevalence of the major non-communicable chronic diseases. These include obesity, type 2 diabetes, cardiovascular disease and many cancers. Group education is likely to provide a better option for scalability when compared to individual one-to-one consultations and may also be more effective through the facilitation of a supporting environment that encourages changes in behaviour.

Published literature demonstrates that group education can provide benefits in terms of knowledge, self-efficacy and health outcomes. Self-management support through the provision of group education, focussing on behaviour change, can help to improve self-efficacy. This in turn can have a positive impact on people's clinical symptoms, attitudes and behaviours, quality of life and patterns of health care resource use. Well-delivered group education, including the peer support, aims to help people learn how to manage their own care more effectively.

There is much to consider when planning and organizing group education. Is the session to be delivered to other healthcare professionals or lay trainers who are going to cascade the information to patient/community groups or is it going to be to the patient/community group themselves? Where is the most appropriate setting to deliver the group? Is it going to be accessible to all those who you are targeting? Does the venue have appropriate facilities? How are you going to meet your overall aim and objectives with the group partici-pants achieving the desired learning outcomes? How are you going to make sure that every group participant is engaged and feels included rather than excluded? What might be different if you are facilitating a group for children rather than adults? How do you make sure that the content and format is appropriate for all groups of society from different ethnic and cultural backgrounds? What resources might be required? There is so much to consider.

This book aims to cover all of these areas so that the facilitator of group education can feel more confident about their approach. It starts by looking at some successful examples of group education, some of the underpinning theory of behaviour change before considering the practical aspects of planning, delivering and evaluating group sessions. The evaluation cannot be overemphasised given the need to prove cost-effectiveness and appropriate use of healthcare resources. Although some people are more naturally effective at facilitating groups and have certain personal qualities, facilitation skills can also be acquired. A good facilitator needs not just to be well prepared but also to be flexible to the needs of an individual group – no two groups are going to behave in the same way! The facilitator needs to be able to think creatively and use a variety of techniques. The effective facilitator does not directly tell people what to do but, instead, provides the nurturing environment whereby they are able to come up with their own personal solutions to maintain optimal long-term health. They are good listeners and skilled at summarizing. They are also good at establishing ground rules for the group.

It is hoped that the reader will find the practice points, top-tips, checklists and practical examples helpful when preparing, facilitating and evaluating groups themselves. We have aimed to include diversity with examples from across the life-course, different settings, different presenting health conditions and different lifestyle changes being targeted. Much of the content is drawn from our own experiences of what we have found most helpful to our practice over the years. We acknowledge that all group facilitators can continue to develop skills and continue to reflect on what went well and what we might do differently next time. We all need to consider our continuing professional development and we hope that this book will be a resource to support that development for all of those who read it.

Acknowledgements

We would like to acknowledge the support of our families during the writing of this book.

We would like to give special thanks to Ruth Stow for reading the draft and offering suggestions for improvements.

Chapter 1 **Introduction**

Amanda Avery

1.1 Overview

This introductory chapter sets the scene explaining why there is a need to find scalable and effective solutions to both prevent and manage the increasing number of non-communicable diseases, such as obesity and type 2 diabetes (T2DM), which result from poor lifestyle habits. Group education, if delivered well, has the potential to provide a solution but the group participant needs to be empowered to feel able to make the desired lifestyle changes. Evidence of successful group education is provided and key characteristics of the successful groups highlighted in the form of 'Top Tips'. These features are then discussed in more detail in subsequent chapters.

1.2 The need for lifestyle change

Non-communicable diseases (NCDs) are the major cause of both mortality and morbidity globally, killing more people each year than all other causes combined. Of the 56 million deaths that occurred in 2012, more than two thirds (68%) were due to NCDs, comprising mainly of cardiovascular diseases, cancers, type 2 diabetes and chronic respiratory disease. Liver disease, resulting from both alcohol abuse and non-alcohol fatty liver disease, is increasingly contributing to this list of NCDs. The combined burden of these conditions is greatest in low and middle income populations, where they impose large avoidable costs in human, social and economic terms. Despite this inequitable distribution in prevalence, much of the human and social impact caused through NCDs could be reduced. This could be by both primary and secondary prevention and through a better understanding of

How to Facilitate Lifestyle Change: Applying Group Education in Healthcare, First Edition.
Amanda Avery, Kirsten Whitehead and Vanessa Halliday.
© 2017 John Wiley & Sons, Ltd. Published 2017 by John Wiley & Sons, Ltd.

cost effective and feasible interventions that acknowledge the socioeconomic determinants of health (WHO, 2014).

NCDs are, in the main, caused by four behavioural risk factors that represent modern day lifestyles:

- tobacco use
- unhealthy diet
- insufficient physical activity/sedentary behaviours
- the harmful use of alcohol (WHO, 2010).

These four behavioural risk factors are discussed in more detail as they are likely to be the focal topics for group education.

Tobacco use

Smoking tobacco and the exposure to second-hand smoke is estimated to cause about 71% of all lung cancers, 42% of chronic respiratory disease and nearly 10% of cardiovascular disease. Smoking also increases the risk of diabetes and premature death (WHO, 2012).

Unhealthy diet (and malnutrition)

The World Cancer Research Fund estimated that 27–39% of the main cancers can be prevented by improving diet, physical activity and body composition (WCRF/AICR, 2007). Approximately 16 million (1.0%) disability-adjusted life years and 1.7 million (2.8%) deaths worldwide are attributed to a low fruit and vegetable consumption (Wang et al., 2014). An adequate intake of fruit and vegetables reduces the risk of cardiovascular diseases, stomach cancer and colorectal cancer (Bazzano et al., 2003; Riboli and Norat, 2003). The consumption of high energy processed foods, high in fats and sugar, increase the risk of obesity compared to low energy dense foods such as fruit and vegetables (Swinburn et al., 2004).

The amount of salt consumed is an important determinant of blood pressure levels and overall cardiovascular risk (Brown et al., 2009). It is estimated that reducing dietary salt intake from the current 9–12 g per day to the globally recommended 5 g for adults would have a significant impact on reducing blood pressure and cardiovascular disease (He and MacGregor, 2009).

Besides the amount of fat in the diet being important, so is the type with the replacement of saturated fats with unsaturated fats considered for many years to be beneficial in reducing risk of coronary heart disease (Hu et al., 1997). A Mediterranean style diet, where the fat is mainly unsaturated, is perceived as being a diet we should aspire to.

Many people have a diet that is too high in free sugars, which can lead to weight gain and poor dental health (SACN, 2015). The main sources of free sugars in our diet include soft drinks, table sugar, confectionery, fruit juices, biscuits, cakes, pastries, puddings and breakfast cereals all of which can be replaced by alternatives with a lower sugar content. The alternatives are also likely to have a healthier overall nutrient profile. Free sugars provide no other important nutrients other than being an energy source. The important relationship between healthy teeth and gums and being able to consume a healthy, varied diet is often overlooked.

Whilst the amount of free sugars in most people's diet is too high, the average intake of dietary fibre is too low in developed countries. Dietary fibre is important for colorectal health and alongside a healthy fluid intake and sufficient physical activity, can help to reduce the prevalence of constipation. In the UK the recommended daily amounts for adults have increased from 18 g/day to 30 g/day (SACN, 2015).

Having an adequate intake of micronutrients is also an important aspect of a healthy balanced diet. Micronutrient deficiencies, for example iron, calcium, iodine and vitamin D, are still common, particularly among vulnerable populations. The European Food and Nutrition Action Plan (2015–2020) aims to reduce the prevalence of anaemia in non-pregnant women of reproductive age by 50%. Group education which ensures that naturally iron rich foods are chosen in the diet will be important to ensure that this target can be achieved in such a large group of women.

People and families with lower incomes (in developed countries), generally have a less healthy diet with a lower intake of fruit and vegetables and a higher intake of processed high energy dense junk foods (McLaren, 2007). Whilst many people may be aware of what a healthy balanced diet includes, there is a need to make this diet more accessible and affordable and attractive as well as to support people to develop the skills and confidence needed to prepare healthier foods.

Insufficient physical activity

Insufficient physical activity is the fourth leading risk factor for mortality (WHO, 2009). People who are insufficiently physically active have a 20–30% increased risk of all-cause mortality compared to those who engage in at least 30 minutes of moderate intensity activity on most days of the week (WHO, 2010). The estimated risk of ischaemic heart disease is reduced by 30%, the risk of T2DM by 27% and the risk of breast and colon cancer by 21–25% through participation in 150 minutes of moderate physical activity each week (WHO, 2010). Additionally, physical activity reduces the risk of stroke, hypertension and depression and, given its key role in energy expenditure, is fundamental to energy balance and thus weight management. In 2010, 23% of adults aged over 18 years were insufficiently active, having less than 150 minutes of moderate intensity physical activity or the equivalent per week

(WHO, 2014). The prevalence of insufficient physical activity actually rises according to the level of country income with higher income countries having more than double the prevalence compared to lower income countries for both men and women. Almost 50% of women in high income countries do not get sufficient physical activity (WHO, 2009).

Alcohol

In 2015 the latest data suggests that the harmful use of alcohol, hazardous and harmful drinking, was responsible for 3.3 million (5.9%) deaths per year worldwide (WHO, 2015). More than half of the deaths occurred as a result of NCDs, including cancers, cardiovascular disease and liver cirrhosis with both morbidity and mortality occurring relatively early in life. In the 20–39-year age-group approximately a quarter of total deaths are alcohol related with more men than women affected. An estimated 5.1% of the global burden of disease, as measured by disability-adjusted life years, is caused by the harmful use of alcohol. Beyond the direct health consequences, the harmful use of alcohol leads to significant social and economic losses to both individuals and the wider society.

The relationship between the risk of these diseases and alcohol is dependent on both the amount and also the pattern of alcohol consumption (Rehm et al., 2010). Low risk patterns of alcohol consumption might actually be beneficial for some population groups.

Besides there being a lack of knowledge about what constitutes a unit of alcohol the additional risks of binge drinking are poorly understood. Similarly, people are generally unaware of the energy contribution that alcohol can make to the diet and this can significantly contribute to obesity levels (Gatineau and Mathrani, 2012).

These lifestyle behaviours lead in turn to five key metabolic/physiological changes:
- raised blood pressure (hypertension)
- overweight/obesity
- hyperinsulinemia
- hyperglycaemia
- hyperlipidaemia.

Raised blood pressure

Globally, raised blood pressure is estimated to cause 12.8% of the total number of deaths and 3.7% of the total disability-adjusted life years. It is a major risk factor for coronary heart disease and ischaemic and haemorrhagic stroke (Lim et al., 2007). In some age-groups, the risk of cardiovascular disease doubles for each incremental increase of 20/10 mmHg of blood pressure

(Whitworth, 2003). Besides coronary heart disease and stroke, other complications attributable to a raised blood pressure include heart failure, peripheral vascular disease, renal impairment, retinal haemorrhage and visual impairment (Williams *et al.*, 2004). The global prevalence of raised blood pressure in adults aged over 25 years was approximately 40% (WHO, 2009) and achieving a 25% relative reduction in the prevalence of raised blood pressure remains a WHO target to help prevent and manage NCDs (WHO, 2014). Some ethnic groups are more prone to hypertension at a younger age than others.

Overweight and obesity

Over the past 30 years, obesity has increasingly become one of the greatest public health concerns reaching epidemic proportions. It has a significant impact on both physical and mental health and well-being with an estimated 93.6 million of global disability-adjusted life years caused by being overweight or obese in 2010 (Lim *et al.*, 2012). Nearly three million people die each year as a result of being overweight or obese but this is likely to be a gross underestimate due to its link with a number of other chronic diseases and the complications resulting from the metabolic disturbances. Mortality rates increase with increasing levels of obesity (PSC, 2009). In many countries, approximately two-thirds of the adult population are either overweight or obese and around a quarter are obese. The prevalence of a high body mass index (BMI) increases with income level of a country, but within countries health inequalities are seen, particularly for women. In a high income country, women from the lowest socioeconomic group have twice as high a prevalence of obesity compared to those in the highest socioeconomic group (WHO Global Database, 2014).

For optimal health, the median BMI for adults should be 21–23 kg/m^2 and the target for individuals should be to maintain a BMI between 18.5 and 24.9 kg/m^2 (WHO, 2014). Again some ethnic minority groups, notably people of South Asian origin, benefit from a lower BMI in the healthy range. People of South Asian and black origin will be more likely to experience metabolic complications such as hypertension and type 2 diabetes once their BMI exceeds 23 kg/m^2 (NICE, 2013).

There are direct links between obesity prevalence and the development of T2DM as outlined next. Similarly links have been observed between obesity and cardiovascular disease risk. A raised BMI increases the risk of cancers of the breast, colon/rectum, endometrium, kidney, oesophagus and pancreas (WCRF/AICR, 2007). Overweight and obesity are also associated with impaired mental health well-being and low self-esteem, infertility, poor pregnancy outcomes, sleep apnoea, osteoarthritis and general mobility problems. Given limited mobility, obese people are less likely to engage in physical activity of moderate to high intensity, which exacerbates the health problems they face.

The prevalence of overweight and obesity in children has also increased since the 1990s. T2DM is now being seen in children as a consequence of this increase and the metabolic changes associated with obesity. Early onset of T2DM is associated with an increased risk of morbidity and mortality during the most productive years of life. Microvascular complications can be present at time of diagnosis. Adolescents with T2DM are also prone to secondary obesity-related complications, including hypertension, non-alcoholic fatty liver disease and metabolic syndrome, all of which are associated with increased cardiovascular risk. The earlier that a person develops T2DM, the earlier and more likely they are to be affected by the associated macro- and microvascular complications. This has a significant impact on the quality of their life (Pinhas-Hamiel and Zeitler, 2007). As with adults, being overweight or obese not only affects the physical health of children but also their psychological health. Children may be bullied because of their weight and the underlying weight stigma present in society can mean that they are less likely to achieve their academic and employment potential (Puhl and Brownell, 2003).

Latest figures suggest that the global prevalence of overweight and obesity in children aged under 5 years has increased from around 5% in 2000 to 6.3% in 2013 (WHO Global Database, 2014). With easy access to energy-dense fast foods and a greater number of indoor based leisure activities that lead to sedentary lifestyles, prevalence levels continue to increase with age. This is causing concern to many government health departments. Again, health inequalities are seen, with children of less educated parents being most affected.

The WHO European Region Health Plan for 2020 promotes a life-course approach to help achieve universal access to affordable, balanced and healthy food for all. Organizations such as Public Health England are committed to supporting the development and implementation of a national childhood obesity strategy (PHE, 2015). This life-course approach will include the importance of good maternal nutrition. There will be more focus on antenatal lifestyle advice given the clear associations between growth *in utero* and early infancy and subsequent health, including risk of childhood obesity and adult cardiovascular risk (Barker, 1995). The health benefits of breastfeeding still need to be promoted with more mothers encouraged to both initiate breastfeeding and also to breastfeed for a longer period so that both the mother and infant can get the full benefits. In developed countries we see differences in breastfeeding rates across different socioeconomic groups and efforts to increase breastfeeding rates need to be targeted to more socially deprived communities where the level of maternal education is lower. Establishing good breastfeeding practice is important alongside the introduction of appropriate solid foods, given that good eating habits are acquired at an early age.

Children, up until a certain age and apart from in a school setting, are dependent on their parents with respect to both access to a healthy diet and opportunities to be physically active. Hence any attempt to promote lifestyle change in children should include parents and, for some cultures, grandparents and the extended family also, as the main agent of change. Generally, a family approach works best.

Hyperinsulinaemia/hyperglycaemia/hyperlipidaemia

These metabolic abnormalities are characteristic precursors of both T2DM and cardiovascular disease. The transition from prediabetes to T2DM in adults is usually a gradual progression that occurs over a period of 5–10 years (Weiss *et al.*, 2005). Fundamental to the development of T2DM is a level of insulin resistance. When the muscle and liver become resistant to the action of insulin, as is often the case in overweight and obese individuals, the pancreas tries to compensate by producing more insulin to maintain normal blood glucose levels and this is characterized by hyperinsulinaemia. When pancreatic function is not able to maintain this level of activity, blood glucose levels gradually rise and in the early stage of declining function this would be associated with impaired glucose tolerance. Whilst obesity is probably the most important cause of insulin resistance, it is not the degree of obesity itself but the distribution of body fat that has the greatest effect. Increased visceral fat and decreased subcutaneous fat deposition are more closely linked to insulin resistance. People with an 'apple-shaped' figure and greater abdominal obesity are more likely to develop metabolic abnormalities compared to those with a more 'pear-shaped' figure. Some ethnic groups are genetically more sensitive to abdominal adiposity and these metabolic changes are seen at a lower BMI and it is recommended that different BMI 'cut off' values are used with different ethnic groups (NICE, 2013).

Insulin resistance and hyperinsulinaemia also impair lipid metabolism and are associated with higher circulating triglyceride and free fatty acid levels and lower levels of circulating HDL-cholesterol, the latter being beneficial in reducing the risks of raised cholesterol levels.

Hence it is appropriate that many government health departments are screening for prediabetes in order to offer public health interventions that prevent or delay the progression to T2DM. These interventions are likely to focus on weight management to reduce both insulin resistance and hyperinsulinaemia and prevent the associated abnormalities seen in lipid metabolism. Approximately one quarter of some adult population groups may be found to have prediabetes, according to the WHO guidelines, on screening (Abraham and Fox, 2013).

Summarizing the need for lifestyle change

As indicated previously, a large proportion of NCDs are both preventable and better managed through the reduction of the four modifiable behavioural risk factors. Healthcare systems should deliver interventions for individuals who either already have NCDs or who are at risk of developing them. Further, the long-term nature of many NCDs requires a comprehensive approach that is not dependent on the time of diagnosis or stage of the condition.

Still the main focus of healthcare for NCDs in many countries remains hospital-based acute clinical care based on a medical model. People with NCDs present at hospitals when cardiovascular disease, cancer, diabetes and chronic respiratory disease have reached the stage of being an acute event or with long-term complications already established. This is a very expensive approach that will not contribute to a significant reduction in the burden of NCDs. It also denies people the health and social benefits of taking care of their condition at an early stage. The prevention and management of NCDs needs to be integrated both into primary healthcare and the acute setting. Gaps in the provision of support for people with NCDs can lead to heart attacks, strokes, renal disease, blindness, peripheral vascular disease, amputations and the late presentation of cancer. It can deny people who have been successfully medically treated to make a full recovery and prevent secondary reoccurrence.

Whilst cardiovascular diseases, cancers, diabetes, chronic respiratory disease and, increasingly, liver disease have been listed as the main NCDs contributing to global ill-health, other chronic conditions such as poor mobility, lower back pain, osteoporosis, functional bowel disorders, dementia and poor mental health are of increasing importance. These chronic conditions all contribute to the individual and societal burden and are likely to further increase in prevalence given the aging population. The same four modifiable behavioural risk factors may also contribute either directly or indirectly to the severity of these conditions and may also be used to improve patient outcomes.

Other long-term conditions where group education may play an important role in helping the individual to better manage their health include type 1 diabetes, coeliac disease, physical disabilities including arthritis and chronic kidney disease.

1.3 Why group education?

The 30% of the UK's population with a long-term condition, including non-communicable disease, accounts for 70% of the current NHS spending. Reducing people's dependence on healthcare professionals and increasing their sense of control and well-being is a more intelligent and effective way of working (de Silva, 2011).

Self-care is defined by the WHO as including 'activities that individuals, families and communities undertake with the intention of enhancing health, preventing disease, limiting illness and restoring health' (WHO, 2002). Self-management support through the provision of group education that focusses on behaviour change can help to improve self-efficacy, which in turn can have a positive impact on people's clinical symptoms, attitudes and behaviours, quality of life and patterns of healthcare resource use (Chih *et al.*, 2010; King *et al.*, 2010; Weng *et al.*, 2010; Sol *et al.*, 2011).

> **Self-efficacy** refers to an individual's belief in their ability to successfully change a certain behaviour and to be able to maintain this behaviour change. Those with high levels of self-efficacy feel confident in their own ability to be able to achieve certain goals.

Group education and peer support programmes aim to help people learn how to manage their own care more effectively, including when to use different healthcare services and resources. Many group education sessions take place in a healthcare setting or in the community but there are also some examples that have been delivered in the workplace, children's centres and schools. This book provides examples of different settings in which group education can be delivered.

Information provision alone is unlikely to be sufficient to motivate sustainable behaviour change and improve clinical outcomes.

General components that have been proven to support self-management include:

- involving people in decision making
- emphasizing problem solving
- promoting healthy lifestyles and educating people about their conditions and how to self-manage
- motivating people to self-manage using targeted approaches and structured information and support
- helping people to monitor their symptoms and know when to take appropriate action
- helping people to manage the social, emotional and physical impacts of their conditions
- providing opportunities to share and learn from other service users with the same condition (de Silva, 2011).

Whilst all of these components can be more efficiently delivered through group delivery, it is the benefits of the wider support in the group setting that allow for the opportunities to share and learn from peers. Groups offer a forum for people, and their family or carers, with any long-term condition to gather and learn together.

A group can be defined as **a gathering or an assembly of people with a common interest**, such as diabetes self-management (Mensing and Norris, 2003). The number of people in a group can vary dependent on a number of factors including the topic, the delivery method, the size of the venue, the facilitators preference and ensuring viability. However, a minimum number of group participants is usually required to maximize the full benefits of group support.

Group attendees and educators have an opportunity to use creative approaches to learning.

1.4 What is the evidence for group education?

Putting aside cost-effectiveness, published literature demonstrates that group education for self-care can provide benefits in terms of knowledge, self-efficacy and health outcomes. Much of the literature has studied the benefits of group education for people with diabetes (Mensing and Norris, 2003). Since the 1970s, supporting people with diabetes in groups to help improve their glycaemic control has been seen as an effective intervention. Today, lifestyle interventions are recommended for preventing T2DM in people at high risk with up to a 58% reduction in risk cited as achievable (NICE, 2012). For those people with diabetes, the use of trained lay educators to facilitate the group is being explored with positive findings (Mandalia *et al.*, 2014).

A number of NCDs, other long-term conditions and innovative evidence-based programmes that have been designed to promote lifestyle change in different population groups and that have measured efficacy, are presented as examples to encourage change in practice:

The ROMEO study for people with type 2 diabetes

Italian people (n = 815), with non-insulin treated diabetes and who had been diagnosed with diabetes for at least 1 year were randomized to either a group or to individual care.

Seven 1-hour group sessions with around 10 participants were held over 2 years with the group education including group work, hands-on activities, problem solving, real-life simulations and role playing.

After 4 years, those attending the group sessions had much better diabetes and cardiovascular management, despite being on similar medications.

Equally, their health behaviours, quality of life and knowledge of diabetes were all significantly better (Trento *et al.*, 2010).

TOP TIP FOR SUCCESSFUL GROUPS

Group facilitators receive training, support with materials and regular supervision.
There is more about role play in Chapter 5.

A peer support diabetes prevention programme

A peer support diabetes prevention programme demonstrated effectiveness of a culturally sensitive programme delivered by trained peers in Turkish- and Arabic- speaking communities in Australia. Ten bilingual peer leaders were recruited via a media release from existing health and social networks (leaders included ethnic workers, interpreters, health promotion workers, teachers), and were trained by diabetes educators over a 2-day period. Each leader recruited 10 participants who attended two lots of 2 hour sessions 1 week apart, with support telephone calls as follow up. Leaders were paid for their training time, recruitment of participants and delivering the sessions. The small group intervention was based on a modified, culturally sensitive training manual and delivered using interactive strategies using culturally sensitive foods. Pedometers were given out as an incentive to increase activity levels.

Three months after the programme the participants mean body weight and waist circumference were both significantly reduced, diabetes knowledge enhanced and lifestyle behaviours significantly improved (Sulaiman *et al.*, 2013).

TOP TIP TO ENSURE A CULTURALLY APPROPRIATE COMMUNITY APPROACH IS USED

Culturally appropriate health education is defined as 'education' that is tailored to the cultural or religious beliefs and linguistic skills of the community being approached, taking into account likely literacy skills (Overland, 1993). It could include adapting established 'health education' to innovative delivery methods, such as using community based health advocates, delivering the information to same gender groups or adapting dietary advice to fit the likely diet of the population group (Hawthorne *et al.*, 2008).

In a 2014 Cochrane review and meta-analysis (Attridge *et al.*, 2014), culturally appropriate diabetes health education in ethnic minority groups was found to result in a 0.2–0.5% reduction in HbA1c and improvements in triglycerides and diabetes knowledge. This is despite ethnic minority groups traditionally being viewed as being hard-to-reach and not accessing traditional diabetes care.

Comparing individual versus group therapy for obesity management

Renjilian *et al.* (2001) investigated whether treatment preference affected weight loss outcomes. In their study, adults with obesity who expressed a clear preference for either individual or group therapy were randomly assigned to either their preferred or their non-preferred option, each delivered over 26 weekly sessions and including behavioural weight management training, for example self-monitoring and goal setting. At the end of the 'treatment' the group therapy produced significantly greater reductions in weight compared to individual therapy. No significant effects were observed for treatment preference suggesting that group therapy produces greater weight loss even amongst adults with obesity who expressed a preference for individual treatment.

TOP TIP: ACKNOWLEDGE THAT SOME PEOPLE WILL FEEL UNCOMFORTABLE ABOUT GOING TO A GROUP BUT WILL ACTUALLY DO BETTER BY GOING TO A GROUP

Some people are nervous about going to groups for the first time. Hence it is really important that they are warmly welcomed. It can be helpful if supporting literature is available explaining what happens in the group and this is provided when the person is first invited to the group. Also, providing the contact details of the group facilitator so that the person can contact the facilitator in advance for further reassurance.

In reality there are very few individuals who would not be better going to a group for support. So be brave and make the group support the first choice.

Group education for couples to reduce their risk of cardiovascular disease

Couples were randomized to a group programme delivered over 16 weeks with a series of six sessions. The sessions addressed nutrition, physical activity and the benefits of a healthy lifestyle, and were delivered by an exercise physiologist and a dietitian. Besides the focus on increasing physical activity levels and improving dietary habits, information about behaviour modification was also included. This covered topics such as barriers to behaviour change, costs and benefits of a healthy lifestyle, goal setting, time and stress management. Although reducing alcohol consumption and cigarette smoking were not the main focus, information on these topics was included consistent with the objective of achieving a healthy lifestyle.

Improvements, particularly in dietary behaviour but also in physical activity levels, were seen in a 1-year follow up when compared to the control group (Dzator *et al.*, 2004).

TOP TIP: PROVIDE IN-BETWEEN GROUP SUPPORT

In-between group mail-outs were used to complement the interactive group sessions. Given the use of technology in modern society, text messages may be an effective alternative or the use of social media where a closed Facebook page could provide the additional support.

TOP TIP: ENCOURAGE PEOPLE TO BRING A FRIEND OR ANOTHER FAMILY MEMBER TO THE GROUP

There can be benefits for the group member bringing along their partner, a friend or other family member.

Self-management group programme for people with arthritis

A self-management group programme for people with arthritis involved pairs of lay leaders, most of whom had arthritis themselves, delivering six weekly sessions with guidance by a manual to ensure consistency in delivery. Topics covered in the programme included exercise, cognitive symptom management, dealing with depression and good nutrition besides information about arthritis, setting realistic goals and communications with healthcare professionals. At four and 12 months follow up, the intervention group of 311 people had a greater self-efficacy, were less depressed and had a greater positive mood, had better dietary, exercise and relaxation habits with the number of visits to the GP decreased by the 12 month follow up (Barlow *et al.*, 2000). The underlying self-efficacy theory used in this programme used four efficacy enhancing strategies; skills mastery, modelling, persuasive communication and re-interpretation of symptoms.

TOP TIP: ROLE MODELS INSPIRE OTHER GROUP MEMBERS; ALL GROUP MEMBERS CAN ENCOURAGE ONE ANOTHER

Modelling is a really useful technique whereby a positive role model, who is successfully managing aspects of their life, serves as a source of inspiration to other group members.

And **persuasive communication** is all about group participants encouraging fellow group members to do just a little bit more than they are currently doing.

TOP TIP: THINK ABOUT WHAT OUTCOME MEASURES WILL BE USED TO MEASURE SUCCESS

Self-efficacy is an important outcome measure to report on. Outcome measures are discussed further in Chapter 2.

Group based 'treatment' for childhood obesity in a community setting

In Finland, children aged 7–9 years were randomized to either a family-based group programme or to routine care involving two individual appointments with a physician. The approach of the family-centred group was based on the principles of behavioural and solution-focussed therapy. The programme emphasized the importance of a healthy lifestyle and the well-being of obese children rather than weight management. Parents were targeted as the main agent for change given their responsibility for making changes happen at home. Most lifestyle changes encouraged were intended for the whole family and any overweight or obese parents attending who wanted to lose weight were encouraged.

The group programme consisted of 15 sessions of 90 minutes' duration over 6 months, held separately for the parents and the child, except for the one where making healthy snacks was the main topic. Each group consisted of seven children and their parents. 'Homework' was given to both parents and children so that they could practice certain skills between sessions. The children's programme was adjusted to the child's cognitive developmental level and thus consisted of functional activities with special themes, for example treasure hunting, to encourage continued participation.

The results showed that the children attending the group programme lost significantly more weight for height compared to routine practice. Attrition from the programme was less than 3%, which shows excellent commitment by the children.

The published paper demonstrating the effectiveness of the group programme provides a clear outline of the content of each session (Kalavainen *et al.*, 2007).

TOP TIP: DIFFERENT APPROACHES WILL BE REQUIRED WHEN WORKING WITH CHILDREN OF DIFFERENT AGES

When developing groups for children it is important to consider the age range. A different style of delivery is required for older children and for older adolescents the approach may be to not include their parents, although up until the age of 16, parental consent should be sought to allow participation in the group.

When working with children (and vulnerable adults), it is important that the group facilitators have the required criminal record checks and appropriate safe-guarding measures have been undertaken.

Workplace health promotion programme

A workplace health promotion programme encouraged employees to engage in healthy lifestyles through various challenges, for example, the healthy weight challenge where participants were encouraged to consider their energy intake and expenditure during the holiday period. As the programme was across a number of sites, a team approach was also used; for example, the Mount Everest fitness challenge, where each team moved a certain distance up a web-based map towards the top of Mount Everest by exercising, meeting the Food Pyramid guidelines and by getting adequate rest. Over a thousand employees participated, (around one-fifth of the total eligible), in the programme for either 1 or 2 years and at the end those who participated had, on average, three fewer days absent from the workplace (Aldana *et al.*, 2005).

TOP TIP: THE WORKPLACE IS AN IDEAL SETTING TO DELIVER GROUP EDUCATION FOR LIFESTYLE CHANGE

The workplace is an excellent setting to deliver group education for lifestyle change. Employers are attracted to the investment given the potential to increase productivity through the improved well-being of the workforce. Absenteeism is costly and reducing absenteeism is a positive outcome.

> **TOP TIP: GROUPS CAN WORK WELL TOGETHER IF A TEAM APPROACH IS ADOPTED**
>
> People generally like challenges but for those who are less keen, a group approach is less threatening. A group can be considered as a team of people who are either competing against other groups or who, as a team, are striving for certain goals.

People with serious mental health illness

People with serious mental health illness are at an increased risk for a number of chronic medical conditions, which the HARP peer-led group programme endeavoured to address (Druss *et al.*, 2010).

The six-session group intervention delivered by trained mental health peer leaders helped participants. Advantages were reported in physical health related quality of life, physical activity levels and medication adherence when compared to usual care. Greater advantages were experienced amongst the subgroup with greater social vulnerability.

> **TOP TIP: A GROUP FACILITATOR NEEDS TO BE SENSITIVE TO INCOME LEVELS AND THE POTENTIAL HIGHER COSTS OF HAVING A HEALTHIER LIFESTYLE**
>
> The diet and physical activity components of the group programme had to be modified to address the high rates of social disadvantage in the population. It is important to be sensitive to income levels and the potential higher costs of having a healthier diet and undertaking physical activity. Having tips on how to eat and be more active on a budget are valuable resources.
>
> Some groups may form their own food cooperatives and make the most of special offers.

We can all learn much from the commercial slimming organizations who successfully deliver weekly groups to large numbers of people who are trying to manage their weight. The group facilitators are all role models who have received training and are passionate about supporting others to be equally successful. There are systems in place to praise the achievements of group members, no matter how small these achievements are, but also persuasive communication to encourage people to do even 'better' if they can. The community approach means that the group influences the discussions based on local community needs.

We acknowledge that there will be some people who will benefit more from individual support. For example, it can be quite difficult to support the underweight person with either T2DM or cardiovascular risk factors in a group setting when everyone else in the group is overweight or obese and would benefit from losing weight. However, these individuals are a smaller group with almost 90% of people with T2DM having a raised BMI.

This book will provide the encouragement and support that healthcare professionals and lay trainers need to help them facilitate effective groups motivating people to make lifestyle changes and better manage their own conditions. For scalable solutions to the increasing health burden associated with non-communicable diseases, good practice needs to be cascaded. There is a need for more people to be trained who are effective at delivering group education.

References

Abraham TM and Fox CS (2013). Implications of rising prediabetes prevalence. *Diabetes Care* 36(8): 2139–2144.

Aldana SG, Merrill RM, Price K, Hardy A and Hager R (2005). Financial impact of a comprehensive multisite workplace health promotion program. *Prev Med* 40: 131–137.

Attridge M, Creamer J, Ramsden M, Cannings-John R and Hawthorne K (2014). Culturally appropriate health education for people in ethnic minority groups with type 2 diabetes mellitus. *Cochrane Database of Syst Rev* 9: CD006424. Available from: DOI: 10.1002/14651858.CD006424.pub3. [Accessed November 2015].

Barker DJ (1995). Fetal origins of coronary heart disease. *BMJ* 311: 171–174.

Barlow JH, Turner AP and Wright CC (2000). A randomised controlled study of the arthritis self-management programme in the UK. *Health Educ Res* 15(6): 665–680.

Bazzano LA, Serdula MK and Liu S (2003). Dietary intake of fruits and vegetables and risk of cardiovascular disease. *Current Atherosclerosis Reports* 5(6): 492–499.

Brown IJ, Tzoulaki I, Candeias V Elliott P (2009). Salt intakes around the world: implications for public health. *Int J Epidemiol* 38: 791–813.

Chih AH, Jan CF, Shu SG and Lue BH (2010). Self-efficacy affects blood sugar control among adolescents with type 1 diabetes mellitus. *J Formos Med Assoc* 109(7): 503–510.

de Silva D (2011). *Helping People Help Themselves*. London: The Health Foundation.

Druss BG, Zhao L, von Esenwein SA, Bona JR, Fricks L, Jenkins-Tucker S *et al.* (2010). The Health and Recovery Peer (HARP) Program: a peer-led intervention to improve medical self-management for persons with serious mental illness. *Schizophr Res* 118: 264–270.

Dzator JA, Hendrie D, Burke V, Gianguilio N, Gillam HF, Beilin LJ (2004). A randomised trial of interactive group sessions achieved greater improvements in nutrition and physical activity at a tiny increase in cost. *J Clin Epidemiol* 57: 610–619.

Gatineau M and Mathrani S (2012). *Obesity and Alcohol: An Overview.* Oxford: National Obesity Observatory.

Hawthorne K, Robles Y, Cannings-John R and Edwards AG (2008). Culturally appropriate health education for type 2 diabetes mellitus in ethnic minority groups. *Cochrane Database of Syst Rev* 16(3): CD006424. Available at: DOI: 10.1002/14651858. CD006424.pub2. [Accessed November 2015].

He FJ and MacGregor GA (2009). A comprehensive review on salt and health and current experience of worldwide salt reduction programmes. *J Hum Hypertens* 23: 363–384.

Hu FB, Stampfer MJ, Manson JE, Rimm E, Colditz GA *et al.* (1997). Dietary fat intake and the risk of coronary heart disease in women. *New Engl J Med* 337: 1491–1499.

Kalavainen MP, Korppi MO and Nuutinen OM (2007). Clinical efficacy of group-based treatment for childhood obesity compared with routinely given individual counselling. *Int J Obesity* 31: 1500–1508.

King DK, Glasgow RE, Toobert DJ, Strycker LA, Estabrookes PA *et al.* (2010). Self-efficacy, problem solving and social-environment support are associated with diabetes self-management behaviours. *Diabetes Care* 33(4): 751–753.

Lim SS, Gaziano TA, Gakidou E, Reddy KS, Farzadfar F *et al.* (2007). Prevention of cardiovascular disease in high-risk individuals in low-income and middle-income countries: health effects and costs. *Lancet* 370(9604): 2054–2062.

Lim SS, Vos T, Flaxman AD, Danaei G, Shibuya K *et al.* (2012). A comparative risk assessment of burden of disease and injury attributable to 67 risk factors and risk factor clusters in 21 regions, 1990–2010: a systematic analysis for the Global Burden of Disease Study 2010. *Lancet* 380(9859): 2224–2260.

Mandalia PK, Stone MA, Davies MJ, Khunti K and Carey ME (2014). Diabetes self-management education: acceptability of using trained lay educators. *Postgrad Med J* 90(1069): 638–642.

Mensing CR and Norris SL (2003). Group education in diabetes: effectiveness and implementation. *Diabetes Spectrum* 16(2): 96–104.

McLaren L (2007). Socioeconomic status and obesity. *Epidemiol Rev* 29(1): 29–48.

NICE (2012). *Type 2 Diabetes: Prevention in People at High Risk.* London: NICE.

NICE (2013). *BMI: Preventing Ill Health and Premature Death in Black, Asian and Other Minority Ethnic Groups.* London: NICE.

Overland JE, Hoskins MJ and McGill DK (1993). Low literacy: a problem in diabetes. *Diabetic Med* (10): 847–850.

Pinhas-Hamiel O and Zeitler P (2007). Acute and chronic complications of type 2 diabetes mellitus in children and adolescents. *Lancet* 369: 1823–1831.

Prospective Studies Collaboration (PSC) (2009). Body-mass index and cause-specific mortality in 900 000 adults: collaborative analyses of 57 prospective studies. *Lancet* 373 (9669): 1083–1096.

Public Health England (2015). Who we are and what we do: Annual Plan 2015/6 [Online]. Available from: www.phe.gov.uk [Accessed May 2016].

Puhl RM and Brownell KD (2003). Psychological origins of weight stigma: toward changing a powerful and pervasive bias. *Obesity Rev* (4): 213–227.

Rehm J, Baliunas D, Borges GLG, Graham K, Irving H *et al.* (2010). The relation between different dimensions of alcohol consumption and burden of disease: an overview. *Addiction* 105: 817–843.

Renjilian DA, Perri MG, Nezu AM, McKelvey WF, Shermer RL and Anton SD (2001). Individual versus group therapy for obesity: effects of matching participants to their treatment preferences. *J Consult Clin Psych* 69(4): 717–721.

Riboli E and Norat T (2003). Epidemiological evidence of the protective effect of fruit and vegetables on cancer risk. *Am J Clinl Nutr* 78(S0): 559–569S.

Scientific Advisory Committee on Nutrition (SACN) (2015). *Carbohydrates and Health* [Online]. Available from: www.gov.uk/government/groups/scientific-advisory-committee-on-nutrition [Accessed May 2016].

Sol BG, van der Graaf Y, van Petersen R and Visseren FL (2011). The effect of self-efficacy on cardiovascular lifestyle. *Eur J Cardiovasc Nurs* 10(3): 180–186.

Sulaiman N, Hadj E, Hussein A and Young D (2013). Peer-supported diabetes prevention program for Turkish- and Arabic-speaking communities in Australia. *ISRN Family Medicine*. Available at: DOI: 10.5402/2013/735359. [Accessed November 2015].

Swinburn BA, Caterson I, Seideli JC and James WPT (2004). Diet, nutrition and the prevention of excess weight gain and obesity. *Public Health Nutr* 7(1A): 123–146.

Trento M, Gamba S, Gentile L, Grassi G, Miselli V *et al.* (2010). Rethink organisation to improve education and outcomes (ROMEO). *Diabetes Care* 33(4): 745–747.

Wang X, Ouyang Y, Liu J, Zhu M, Zhao G, Bao W and Hu FB (2014). Fruit and vegetable consumption and mortality from all causes, cardiovascular disease, and cancer: systematic review and dose-response meta-analysis of prospective cohort studies. *BMJ* 349: g4490.

Weng IC, Dai YT, Huang HL and Chiang YJ (2010). Self-efficacy, self-care behaviours and quality of life of kidney transplant recipients. *J Adv Nurs* 66(4): 828–838.

Weiss R, Taksali SE, Tamborlane WV, Burgent TS, Savoye M and Caprio S (2005). Predictors of change in glucose tolerance status in obese youth. *Diabetes Care* 28: 902–909.

Whitworth JA (2003). World Health Organisation/International Society of Hypertension statement on the management of hypertension. *J Hypertens* 21: 1983–1992.

WHO (2002). *Innovative Care for Chronic Conditions. Building Blocks for Action.* Geneva: World Health Organisation.

WHO (2009). *Global Health Risks: Mortality and Disease Attributable to Selected Major Risks.* Geneva: World Health Organisation.

WHO (2010). *Global Recommendations on Physical Activity for Health.* Geneva: World Health Organisation.

WHO (2012). *WHO Global Report. Mortality Attributable to Tobacco.* Geneva: World Health Organisation.

WHO (2014). *Global Status Report on Noncommunicable Diseases 2014: Attaining the Nine Global Noncommunicable Disease Targets; A Shared Responsibility.* Geneva: World Health Organisation.

WHO (2015). *Alcohol Factsheet* [Online]. Available at: www.who.int/mediacentre/factsheets/fs349/en/ [Accessed May 2016].

Williams B, Poulter NR, Brown MJ, Davis M, McInnes GT *et al.* (2004). British Hypertension society guidelines for hypertension management summary. *BMJ* 328: 634–640.

World Cancer Research Fund/American Institute for Cancer Research (WCRF/AICR) (2007). *Food, Nutrition, Physical Activity and the Prevention of Cancer: A Global Perspective.* Washington DC: AICR.

Chapter 2 **Behaviour change**

Kirsten Whitehead

2.1 Introduction

This chapter will consider what we mean by behaviour change in the context of a healthy lifestyle and group education. Although there are many ways that health related behaviour change can be supported, including environmental change, taxation on unhealthy products, changes in food production (e.g. decreasing salt content of foods), the focus will be on what can be done within the context of group education. There is a huge literature on behaviour change with many theoretical models and a comprehensive overview of these can be found in Michie *et al.* (2014a). Some theories and models will be described to illustrate how they can help when planning and evaluating group education. Facilitators need to understand the factors that affect the behaviour of the participants in order to design group education that is most likely to support change. Specific examples of behaviour change techniques that can be either used or taught within the group education setting will be discussed, including goal setting, action planning, social support, self-monitoring and use of rewards.

2.2 What is behaviour change?

So what do we mean by behaviour change? Behaviour is the way that people act or conduct themselves and the actions they take or don't take, which includes their interaction with others. Therefore, behaviour change is about changing the way people act and what they do. In the context of health that relates to the way an individual changes their behaviour towards a healthier lifestyle, for example stopping smoking, decreasing alcohol consumption to a healthy level, replacing unhealthy snacks with healthier options, replacing

---

a sedentary activity with an active one and so on. Group education therefore needs to be designed to include specific activities that will support the health related behaviour change required by the aim of the session. If the aim is weight management, then the content must support changes in behaviour that will lead to decreased energy intake and/or increased physical activity. A smoking cessation service must be designed to support participants to stop smoking. However, it is important to consider that there may be many different actions that support that overall change. For example, with the smoking cessation this could include using nicotine replacement therapies, identifying and using healthy alternative activities to take place of the smoking, implementing alternative ways of managing stress and so on. It is not usually one action or change in behaviour that leads to meeting the aim of the group education. Similarly, individual participants will have different actions to take to meet that behaviour change. Two overweight participants may have completely different dietary and physical activity patterns and therefore the specific changes will need to be different as will the way the individual goes about putting that change into action. As a facilitator, this is really important to understand.

2.3 Why is behaviour change so important for lifestyle change?

The importance of lifestyle change has been outlined in Chapter 1 and is clearly needed globally to decrease the incidence, morbidity and mortality and the huge economic burden related to NCDs. Many people are aware that lifestyle change could decrease their risk of these diseases and improve their health but they do not translate that into action. Health promoters have been working to try and educate individuals and populations to improve lifestyle for decades but still unhealthy lifestyles are having a huge impact. There is a gap between knowing that there needs to be change and this change actually happening. What appears to be 'common sense', for example smoking is unhealthy therefore everyone should stop smoking, does not translate to everyone making that change in behaviour. Why is that? This is where our understanding of behaviour change fits and in recent years there have been developments in the science and evidence to support this.

2.4 Behaviour change theory and models

Behaviour change theories or models are designed to help us clarify why, when and how behaviour does or does not occur. They also help to identify what is influencing behaviour and therefore areas that could be targeted in order to support behaviour change (Michie *et al.*, 2014a). They can help us understand and perhaps explain what is going on and are important when planning interventions (NICE, 2007). As more knowledge is gained about human behaviour and what affects it, theory is in constant need of being developed and refined (Michie *et al.*, 2014a). A theory must provide an explanation for what is being observed and should allow for the prediction of behaviour. It should also include reference to internal factors such as physiological and physical factors about the individual, but also external factors such as the environment or social networks that the individual is part of.

There are many behaviour change theories and it is likely that many group education facilitators will be aware of some, but not all of these. Some that have been commonly used in the area of health promotion include the Health Belief Model (Becker, 1974), The Transtheoretical Model of Behaviour Change (Prochaska and DiClemente, 1982), which has commonly been used in the area of addictive behaviour and smoking cessation, and the Theory of Planned Behaviour (Ajzen, 1991). A comprehensive overview of behaviour change theories is provided by Michie *et al. (2014a)*.

It is also difficult when looking at lifestyle modification, as there are so many different aspects of lifestyle that may benefit from behaviour change. It is unlikely that any individual attending group education would benefit from making only one change to their behaviour. In practice, many interventions use integrated approaches to behaviour change that include elements from different models or theories. Many behaviour change models have been highly criticized because they don't include a complete understanding of human behaviour. For example, many do not include issues such as habit, self-control or the impact of emotion. All of these are extremely relevant when looking at behaviours such as food intake, physical activity, smoking and alcohol consumption. NICE (2007) concluded that the evidence base did not support the use of one particular behaviour change model but training of healthcare professionals to support behaviour change was identified as a priority. Table 2.1 shows useful questions to help guide the planning of behaviour change interventions (NICE, 2007) and this can be applied to group education. These should be considered right at the beginning of the planning process.

More recently, a framework for understanding behaviour, Capability, Opportunity, Motivation-Behaviour (COM-B) has been developed (Michie *et al.*, 2011) and this can be very helpful when planning group education interventions. This is shown diagrammatically in Figure 2.1.

Capability refers to the individual's capability to engage with the behaviour change suggested. This is from a psychological point of view, which includes

Table 2.1 Questions to guide the planning of behaviour change interventions. Source: Adapted from NICE (2007).

Whose health are you seeking to improve (target population/s)?

What behaviour are you seeking to change (behavioural target)?

What contextual factors need to be taken into account (what are the barriers to and opportunities for change and what are the strengths/potential of the people you are working with)?

How will you know if you have succeeded in changing behaviour (what are your intended outcomes and outcome measures)?

Which social factors may directly affect the behaviour and can they be tackled? (For example, income or cultural issues.)

What assumptions have been made about the theoretical links between the intervention and outcome? (Model of behaviour change.)

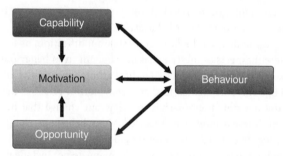

Figure 2.1 The COM-B system.

their ability to comprehend and apply reasoning, but is also about having the physical capacity to engage. Capability includes having necessary knowledge and skills, which is part of what a group education intervention can provide. For example, providing group participants with an understanding of the physical activity recommendations and information on where to access some physical activity opportunities could increase their capability to improve their physical activity level, but only if they have the physical capacity to undertake those activities. The group facilitator will need to ensure that they consider the physical capacity of group participants. A participant who is a wheelchair user will not improve their capability by being given information on the physical activity recommendations and how to use a pedometer. In this case, the information or knowledge needs to be related to the physical capacity of that participant and possibly include skill development by teaching about physical activities that they have physical capacity to undertake. With food intake, it may be that skills need to be acquired by group participants to purchase healthy food within a budget or to develop cooking skills. Increasing the capability of participants may improve their motivation as behaviour change may be perceived as more achievable to them.

Opportunity refers to factors that are external to the individual participants and make behaviour change possible. They may also act as a prompt or a reminder to participants. Group education sessions in themselves are an opportunity for group participants. They may provide knowledge and skills, for example cooking skills, problem-solving ability or social support, which make it possible for participants to engage in a healthier behaviour. Both capability and opportunity will influence motivation.

Motivation is a combination of all factors that energize and direct our behaviour choices. It is not just goals to set or conscious decisions but includes our habits, emotions and ability to make decisions. For a facilitator of group education, developing and using motivational interviewing skills can help group participants to become more aware of their internal motivating factors. Motivational interviewing can also help participants to resolve ambivalence; that is, when they have simultaneous but conflicting feelings about a course of action. Often ambivalence means that the individual continues with unhealthy behaviour because they cannot decide on a way forward. Therefore, ambivalence can be a significant barrier to behaviour change. A skilled facilitator will be able to identify this with individual participants and may be able to support them towards healthier behaviour change. If the facilitator has not been trained in motivational interviewing they can still motivate participants by using active listening skills and demonstrating empathy.

Motivational interviewing skills are discussed further in Chapter 3. Further information about these skills, evidence base and training opportunities can be found at www.motivationalinterviewing.org/.

2.5 Behaviour change interventions

What do we mean by the phrase 'behaviour change intervention'? This has been described as 'sets of techniques, used together, which aim to change the health behaviours of individuals, communities or whole populations' (NICE, 2014). Group education usually focusses on the individual participants and individual-level behaviour change interventions have been described as those that 'aim to help someone with a specific health condition or a behaviour that may affect their health' (NICE, 2014). Michie *et al.* (2011) describe behaviour change interventions as coordinated sets of activities that are designed to change specific behaviour patterns.

Developing behaviour change interventions

When planning a behaviour change intervention, facilitators will need to consider what the behavioural target is going to be, what would need to be changed in order to meet that target and how might they go about achieving the behaviour change with the target participants. A key focus is on creating a 'measurable' change in a specific person or group of people such as a change in energy intake, which is significant enough to lead to weight loss or stopping binge drinking of alcohol and moving to drinking within the recommended levels. In group education you could measure a variety of behaviours, such as how many of the participants are now smoking, how many have lost weight, average weight loss across the group, self-efficacy in relation to making healthy decisions, how many participants have moved from being sedentary to meeting physical activity guidelines and so on. What to measure is discussed in more detail in Chapter 7 on evaluation. Michie *et al.* (2014b) describe detailed information on factors that influence behaviour, intervention options and evaluation processes.

Behaviour change interventions should be clearly described so they can be reliably replicated. However, many in the literature lack detail (NICE, 2014). Davidson *et al.* (2003) described the minimal detail that should be described in research papers or intervention reports and this is applied to group education in Table 2.2. Facilitators should consider from the very beginning the need to present the results of the education to stakeholders or to wider audiences. For other facilitators to learn from the work this level of detail needs to be made available.

2.6 Behaviour change techniques

Behaviour change techniques are the specific parts of a behaviour change intervention that are designed to change behaviour, for example social support, goal setting, action planning, self-monitoring, rewards, distraction and so on. These should be very clearly described so that facilitators understand what is being done and why. One of the difficulties with interpreting published literature about lifestyle change interventions is that these techniques are often very poorly described and it is therefore very difficult to work out which technique it was that led to a behaviour change (Michie *et al.*, 2013). A clearly specified intervention is an essential prerequisite to meaningful evaluation.

Table 2.2 Detail required when describing interventions.

Intervention component	Intervention question addressed	Example
Content and delivery method	What was the content of the intervention and how was it delivered?	What? Safe alcohol intake and ways to decrease alcohol consumption. How? Oral presentation, video and group activities to identify alcohol and energy content of different drinks and to support participants to accurately estimate weekly alcohol consumption. Written resources to take away to reinforce messages given including current recommendations for alcohol consumption.
Provider	Who delivered it?	Health promotion practitioner specializing in alcohol use and misuse.
Format	What method of intervention administration was used? For example, telephone, individual consultation, group session	Group education session.
Setting	Where and when was the intervention delivered?	Local health centre.
Recipient	To whom was the intervention delivered? Was the recipient also the target of the intervention?	Overweight and obese patients at risk of CHD who have been identified as consuming alcohol above the safe levels.
Intensity	How many different contacts and how much total contact time was involved?	1 × 2-hour session as part of a series of 6 sessions on weight management
Duration	Over what time period were the intervention contacts undertaken and how were they spaced?	Full programme over 10 weeks with one session every 2 weeks

(Continued)

Table 2.2 Continued

Intervention component	Intervention question addressed	Example
Fidelity	Was the intervention delivered as intended? How was this monitored and measured?	Health promotion practitioner was off sick and session was facilitated by the practice nurse. Debrief with team leader suggested that the programme was followed but the practice nurse added in some anecdotes in the presentation to illustrate the points and make it more interesting.

Goal setting

Goal setting theory was developed in industrial and organizational psychology over many years (Locke and Latham, 2006) but has been applied to the health setting. It explains how goals can affect performance in defined tasks and how that performance can be influenced by level of commitment, the importance of the goal to the individual, the level of self-efficacy of the individual, what feedback they receive and the complexity of the goal set (Michie *et al.*, 2014a). A goal is an action with a measurable result, often with a date by which it will be achieved (Cullen *et al.*, 2001). In the health-care setting, collaborative goal setting is seen as a process by which caregiver and patient (or facilitator and participant) agree on a health-related goal with a concrete course of action to move the patient/participant toward that goal (Bodenheimer and Handley, 2009). In some cases, the word **target** is used and is understood to mean the same in this context. Goal setting has been recognized and used as a behaviour change technique and a core component of diabetes care leading to improvements in self-efficacy, food intake, physical activity levels and blood glucose control (Miller and Bauman, 2014). There are still questions to be answered about when and how it is most effective but it is well accepted that goal setting is a useful behaviour change technique. In a group education setting, the facilitator will support each participant to set their own goals as these will need to be individualized, but the way that it is done may be as a group or individual activity.

Cullen *et al.* (2001) outlined a four-step process, which is explained in detail next:

1 Recognize the need for change
2 Establish a goal
3 Monitor goal related activity
4 Reward yourself for goal attainment.

Recognizing the need for change

Facilitators need to include within the group education session an opportunity for participants to gain clear information about why the behaviour change is needed. This might include a summary of evidence for the benefits in everyday language; for example, of stopping smoking, avoiding sedentary behaviour, eating a healthier diet and so on. It is really important to talk about this carefully and positively to avoid participants feeling judged for not having a perfect lifestyle. It is better to focus on what participants will gain by making changes rather than on all of the dangers and risk of their current lifestyle. It is not uncommon for participants to be misinformed or simply not know why a change in lifestyle is important for their health. Participants may not realize how overweight they are in comparison to the recommendations for a healthy body mass index (BMI), or how unhealthy their diet is, or how little physical activity they do in comparison to the recommendations. Many people are unaware of the energy content of alcoholic drinks and, as well as the risks associated with excessive alcohol consumption, the fact that alcohol may be contributing significantly to their energy intake and consequently weight. Even if participants are aware of the details of health recommendations, they may be unable to translate them to their own lifestyle. An example of this is that many people are aware of the number of portions of fruit and vegetables they should eat per day, but do not know what counts as a portion. Many people do not possess food weighing scales and cannot therefore weigh foods in the home environment, so handy measures are going to be essential to help them work out how many portions they are currently consuming. Facilitators should not assume that participants will be well informed in relation to health recommendations. On the contrary it is likely that the knowledge within the group will be variable and that some participants will be surprised or shocked when they realize the possible consequences of their lifestyle. There can sometimes be emotional reactions to this increasing awareness and the facilitator should be aware of this possibility and prepared to offer support if required. Chapter 3 covers the facilitator skills and discusses further how to support participants in these situations.

Establishing a goal

Once the participants have recognized the need for change they can move on to establishing a goal. However, it is important for facilitators to check if the participants have reached the point of wanting to change their lifestyle. If they haven't, then they will not be committed to the goal and it is therefore important to explore why that is. It may be that the participant still does not recognize the need for them personally to change, they might require more information such as how food relates to their medical condition and therefore what effects the change in food intake will have. This might be particularly important with participants who have diabetes, hypertension or hyperlipidaemia. Participants may not believe that they are capable of making changes (i.e. have a low self-efficacy). They may not be able to see a way forward for them and so are reluctant to set a goal through fear of failing to achieve it. The facilitator has the challenging job of working with a group with the same overall aim but whose individual goals may be quite different to each other.

The development of goals needs to be participant-centred, individualized and with active participation (NICE, 2012). It is really important the facilitators do not try to persuade or force participants to set goals that they are not comfortable with. It is common to start with small easy changes which, when met, build self-efficacy. Short term or proximal goals can help get a participant started on a behaviour change if the long term goal is too difficult for the participant. However, more difficult (but achievable) goals can lead to greater effort as long as the goals are clear and specific. Goals are well recognized as being motivational and this is more so when an individual freely makes a decision and feels responsible for it (Cullen *et al.*, 2001). Health promoting goals can direct behaviour away from unhealthy alternative behaviours. The facilitator needs to guide participants to goals that are relevant to the aim of the lifestyle change. Table 2.3 summarizes some examples of aims, goals and action plans to support behaviour change.

Monitoring goal-related activity

Although facilitators may undertake some monitoring, for example regular weighing in a weight management group, this mostly refers to self-monitoring. There are many ways in which participants can monitor their own progress in relation to the goals set.

In relation to food intake, participants may focus on a specific area, for example fruit and vegetable intake, and keep a record of how many portions they consume a day, they may keep a food diary or use an app on their phone, iPad or tablet. Participants may record what, where, when and how much they eat as well as the situation or circumstances they were in, for example

Table 2.3 Health-related goals and action plans.

Aim	Goal	Action plan
Weight loss	To lose 3 kg in the next month	In order to prepare for the healthier lifestyle, the following tasks need to be completed: • On Monday, sign up for cook and eat classes to learn how to cook healthy family meals. • Before Monday, plan meals for the week in advance and make shopping list based on that. Stick to the list! • From tomorrow, keep a food and activity diary for 1 week to identify patterns and where unhealthy high energy foods are being consumed. • Identify what snacks are being consumed and plan and purchase lower energy alternatives. • Investigate the facilities for bicycles at work. Work out a safe route to work. Buy a cycle helmet. Clean the bike and ensure it is roadworthy. From the following week: • Limit takeaway meals to once a week (planning meals will help facilitate this). • Alternate alcoholic drinks with sugar-free soft drinks (warn partner in advance that this is going to happen). • Limit unhealthy snacks to twice a week. Plan when they are going to be consumed. • Start cycling to work on Tuesdays and Thursdays.
Stop smoking	Quit by the end of next month	This week: • Access Nicotine Replacement Therapy. • Keep a diary of the times when I smoke, what I am doing and how I am feeling. • Plan how to distract myself from wanting a cigarette. • Buy sugar-free mints. • Develop a strategy for coping when with friends who are still smoking. • Write a list of activities that help with relaxation and stress management. • Enlist the support of non-smoking friends and family. Next week: • Stop smoking on Monday • Keep diary of how it is going, what is difficult and how I deal with it. • Attend group.

attending a work event where lunch was provided or a meal out with friends. This can help people to identify the occasions and situations where they find it difficult to follow their dietary recommendations.

With physical activity participants can keep an activity diary where they record what type of activity and how long they undertook it for. They may use a pedometer or other activity monitoring tools such as a Fitbit™ or phone app. Again, they may want to record the circumstances that affected what they were doing such as 'didn't go for my walk this morning as it was raining really hard' or 'my appointment was cancelled and I had time on my hands so I went swimming'.

Similar tools are available to help people monitor the number of units of alcohol consumed and diaries can be used for smoking. Participants may be monitoring specific behaviours that they have been trying to change, for example, automatically eating a biscuit with a cup of coffee or sitting for long periods of time. In some cases, monitoring clinical outcomes such as blood glucose levels, body weight or blood pressure can be undertaken either by the participant or by a health professional.

It is important not to be prescriptive about how people monitor their progress as not everyone will have access to each type of monitoring tool and people may have strong preferences for one method or another. It has been found in many cases that self-monitoring is more effective than being monitored by another person such as a healthcare professional in the long term. For example, Reyes *et al.* (2012) found that people who lost weight and maintained that weight loss over time were more likely to self-monitor, including weighing themselves regularly. One of the advantages of monitoring progress is that it gives immediate feedback. Feedback is known to influence performance towards a goal as knowing how you are progressing allows people to adjust their strategies or amount of effort if they are not progressing as planned. Knowing that you are attending another group education session where your progress may be questioned can help to keep people focussed. However, not progressing well may be an explanation for people failing to return. The facilitator needs to make it clear that failing to achieve goals is common and requires a problem solving approach, which can be supported in the group setting. Participants need to be reassured that they are welcome and encouraged to attend whether they have progressed well or not. If participants feel judged for not achieving a goal they are not likely to want to return to the group. Some participants will be very tough on themselves if they have failed to meet a goal. A positive, encouraging approach that helps them to understand what went wrong, along with problem solving, will help the participant to start afresh. Pearson and Grace (2012) provide more detail on self-monitoring in relation to weight management.

Rewards for goal attainment

For some people, reaching a goal is highly satisfying and the sense of achievement is a reward in itself. It can be helpful in the group setting to come up with ideas on suitable rewards, bearing in mind that personal preferences and resources will be very different. If the behaviour change has been food related, then going out for a meal is probably not the best option. Having suitable rewards planned in advance can be useful as it can give participants something to look forward to. Rewards have to be based on what matters to the individual. As a group facilitator, it is important to give praise and congratulations to participants; that in itself can be perceived as a reward.

TOP TIPS: REWARDS FOR GOAL ATTAINMENT

- Have an activity in the session where participants decide upon and record what will be a suitable reward for them. Some sharing of ideas amongst the group can be helpful but the specific rewards will be an individual choice.
- If participants are stopping smoking or cutting down alcohol consumption they may wish to put aside some of the money saved for something special to them, for example a night out, attendance at a sporting event, a weekend away, new clothes or a gift for someone special to them.
- Praise goal attainment. For some people that is a reward that they will value.
- Support those who have not attained their goal and help them work out what went wrong and a new strategy to support future goal attainment.
- If running a series of sessions, it may be possible to have some rewards to offer those who have achieved the most that can act as an incentive, for example high street vouchers.

Action planning

This links closely with goal setting as it is about deciding on a course of action that will lead to the goal being met. An action plan includes a description of events relating to the goals such as what will happen in specific situations, what time frame it will happen in, how long it will go on and where it will take place.

When is the participant going to start working towards their goal? It is easy to think that the participant should start immediately. However, there may be very valid reasons for waiting. For example, if a participant is making dietary changes towards a healthier lifestyle but is about to go on holiday where all food is provided, it may be difficult for them to control their eating behaviour. It may be better to set small targets to reduce the chance of weight gain on holiday rather than trying to implement significant change at that time.

They may decide that they can limit additional snacks that they may typically have on holiday, such as ice cream or cake, rather than changing the meals provided for them. Similarly, if they are going away with a group of people who all smoke it may be difficult for that individual to stop smoking. Understanding the participant scenario is essential to help them to set a realistic start date. In contrast, some participants may constantly come up with reasons why they should not start making changes and may need encouragement to start somewhere.

What needs to be in place? There may be a need for skill development to support the participant to change their behaviour. They may need to develop their cooking skills to support a healthier diet, obtain nicotine replacement therapy prior to stopping smoking or to buy suitable shoes to enable them to go on longer walks. Again, there needs to be a balance between being realistic about what participants can do and supporting participants to overcome perceived barriers.

Table 2.3 gives some examples of health-related goals and possible action plans to achieve them. Both goals and action plans need to be reviewed regularly to assess progress: Has the goal been met? Is the action plan working? Is there a need to change either the goal or the action plan? There may be several actions that are designed to move the participant towards the goals.

Stimulus control

For many people there are particular situations or emotions that tend to lead to unhealthy behaviours. These are often referred to as **triggers** or **stimuli**. Participants can be supported within group education to identify situations where they personally are most likely to be tempted to undertake unhealthy behaviour. Often some group participants are willing to share the situations that they find difficult and this can be really helpful to encourage other participants. The group scenario can be very supportive as people realize that they are not on their own and other people have similar experiences. Facilitating a group activity that encourages some level of sharing and then moves the participants to problem-solving and learning how to control stimuli or triggers requires empathy with the participants and a non-judgemental attitude. Table 2.4 identifies some common triggers or stimuli for unhealthy behaviours alongside some possible strategies. As with goals needing to be individualized, stimuli and triggers are very much individual as are the strategies that will be needed to control them. For example, some people will prefer not to have alcohol or an unhealthy food in their home because they know if it is there they will struggle to avoid consuming it. That may be difficult if there are other people who will be

Table 2.4 Examples of common triggers for unhealthy behaviour and possible strategies.

Trigger	Possible strategies
Stress or anxiety	Relaxation techniques Social support
Boredom	Prepared list of activities and tasks that the individual wishes to achieve Social support
Social engagements	Offer to drive (and therefore do not drink alcohol) Eat healthy food before going to avoid overconsumption of unhealthy food Where feasible, suggest alternative healthier types of social activity, e.g. a walk in the countryside with a picnic (where the individual can control what food they eat) rather than meeting in the pub for a drink and pub lunch where it will be tempting to eat and drink more Social support

affected by that decision. In that case it may be that the participant needs to have those items out of their sight rather than out of the home.

Distraction

With some types of behaviour participants will need to overcome their habits and craving, for example with food, alcohol and smoking.

With food, participants may experience cravings; that is, an urge to eat that is not hunger. In many cases, participants will find themselves faced with the sight and smell of food constantly throughout the day and it is difficult to block the thought of food and desire for food out of your mind. It is also common for people to strongly desire or crave foods that they have decided they are not going to eat. Distraction is one behavioural technique that can be very helpful. Cravings or urges to eat usually last about 15–20 minutes (Pearson and Grace, 2012). Distracting yourself until that urge or craving has passed is an active process and suitable distractions can be planned in advance. These may include activities such as phoning a friend, writing a letter, cleaning or tidying something, doing something active like going for a walk, gardening or some other activity that requires your full attention and does not involve eating. Having a list of such activities including tasks that the participant would actually like to achieve, and can then tick off when they have achieved them, will work for some people and can be motivating. Not only did they avoid the unhealthy behaviour but they actually achieved something positive at the same time. Relaxation techniques can help people to overcome unhealthy behaviours that are undertaken as a result of stress or anxiety. Many similar activities can be used to support participants to avoid having a cigarette or another alcoholic drink; however, they may also wish to avoid putting themselves in situations where they are likely to be tempted or offered these things.

Within group education, the facilitator may ask group participants to share what might work for them as individuals to increase the number of ideas. Individual participants can then create their own lists with distractions that they think will work for them.

Social support

Social support is the comfort, caring, esteem or help a person receives from other individuals or groups that they have contact with. Sarafino (2014) described three different types of social support:

1 **Emotional**. This relates to how cared for or esteemed a person feels by the people around them.
2 **Tangible**. This is sometimes described as instrumental support and can be very practical, such as going to an activity with the participant or helping them to make plans.
3 **Informational**. Knowledge and information that is related to the required lifestyle change.

Some of this support can be provided by the group education itself. One of the roles of the healthcare professional is to provide accurate evidence-based information. As well as the facilitator, group members may often provide emotional support for each other and share ideas of how to support health behaviour change. However, for some there will be a need for social support external to the group such as friends or family members. It is important for the facilitator and other group members not to make the assumption that a participant will receive support outside of the group. This again is an area that needs to be handled carefully as in some cases partners or family may make it more difficult for the participant to make healthy behaviour changes. The facilitator may wish to ask if participants can identify sources of social support outside of the group. For some participants this may be more diffi-cult than others. There may be other sources of support such as self-help groups and some of these will be online as opposed to a group of local people who meet together. As a facilitator, it is important to be aware of local groups or online groups that may provide support for participants.

Do also consider that some people who are expected to provide social sup-port may do exactly the opposite. The ways in which an individual wishes to be supported may be different to how those around them are trying to support them. A facilitator can help group participants to identify what is helpful for them and what is not. This may empower participants to be clear with their supporters about what works best for them.

Visualization

Visualization is a technique that involves participants focussing on positive mental images in order to support them to achieve a particular goal. In the group setting an activity could be to give participants a few minutes to close their eyes and focus on where they wish to be in a certain time frame, for example 3 months. For example, a participant who is trying to lose weight might visualize themselves getting back into a favourite item of clothing that is not currently big enough for them. Participants may be able to imagine themselves behaving differently in particular social situations, for example enjoying a social event without getting drunk or having to go outside for a cigarette. This process is in effect another form of goal setting but having a clear visual picture may be more helpful for some participants.

There are many other behaviour change techniques that can be incorporated into group education and a detailed description of these can be found in Michie et al. (2013).

Communication skills as a tool for behaviour change

The communication skills of the facilitator are discussed in Chapter 3 and these will have a profound effect on the desire and ability of the participants to implement behaviour change. Building and maintaining rapport, active listening skills and appropriate questions will all contribute to the support that participants need in order to make changes in behaviour. Good communication skills may also help when participants are problem solving and trying to find ways to overcome the barriers that they face.

Barriers to behaviour change

For many participants, there will be a range of factors that influence their ability and willingness to change their behaviour. A good facilitator will recognize these and work with participants to find ways around them. As facilitators work with different groups and become more experienced, they will become more familiar with what to be aware of. There are many barriers that will influence a variety of lifestyle factors and some that will be specific, for example to food intake and dietary change. Table 2.5 provides a list of commonly occurring factors that can act as barriers to participant behaviour change.

Table 2.5 Common barriers to behaviour change.

Lifestyle factor	Common barriers
General changes to healthier lifestyle	Likes and dislikes, personal preferences. Time. Busy lifestyles get in the way of people having time to think through and plan for lifestyle change. Lack of knowledge about healthier alternatives. Lack of self-efficacy; i.e. the participant does not believe that they will be able to make and sustain change. Many people live their lives in similar ways to their parents and perceive that that is the right way rather than ever questioning that. Habits can be difficult to change. Social pressure from family, friends or work colleagues. Culture (can be a positive or negative influence). Lack of social support. Lack of health literacy, that is, the degree to which people have the capacity to obtain, process and understand basic health information and services needed to make appropriate health decisions (Parker *et al.*, 2003).
Healthy diet	Lack of shopping facilities/access to healthier foods. Poor transport facilities. Cost/affordability of healthy foods. Unfamiliarity and negative perceptions of healthy foods. Long or irregular work hours such as shift work. Poor facilities or access to healthy food in the work environment. Lack of cooking facilities and/or equipment. Healthy foods can often be perishable and could potentially lead to more food waste, which is costly. Some healthy alternatives may require lengthier preparation and busy people may be looking for convenience rather than healthy alternatives. Lack of storage space. Not having control of what food is purchased and prepared within the home. Lack of knowledge and skills for budgeting, shopping and cooking. Lack of knowledge about food and health. No desire to change eating habits. Confusing or inconsistent messages about what a healthy diet consists of. Poor literacy affecting ability to read and understand food labels and food information. Health problems including sore mouth, poor dentition, nausea, swallowing difficulties, gastro-intestinal problems, poor appetite. Physical disabilities such as visual impairment or poor mobility. Some medications increase appetite. Mental health problems such as depression or anxiety, stress and trauma. Use of recreational drugs can lead participants to have a very sweet tooth and crave sweet foods, have a chaotic lifestyle and lack of available income for healthier food.

(Continued)

Table 2.5 (Continued)

Lifestyle factor	Common barriers
Physical activity	Cost-including appropriate clothing and/or shoes, equipment (e.g. bicycles, badminton rackets, cycle helmets), gym membership and costs of activity classes. Lack of access to physical activity opportunities such as parks, leisure centres, swimming pools, gyms, activity classes. Lack of safe places to walk or cycle or fear for safety. Lack of knowledge about physical activity opportunities available. Lack of understanding of everyday activities that count as physical activity, such as housework, gardening and active travel. Embarrassment about being seen undertaking physical activity. Effort required both physically and with organization. Health reasons such as poor mobility, asthma, chronic obstructive pulmonary disease. Lack of confidence in ability to undertake specific physical activities; for example, for those who are not well coordinated undertaking activities that require coordination. For those who are overweight or obese there are risks of discomfort such as friction burns. Lack of suitable machinery (in gyms) for heavier participants. Lack of childcare.
Smoking cessation	Lack of self-efficacy in relation to stopping smoking. This may be particularly if previous attempts have failed. Smoking may be a coping mechanism for stress. Participants may fear stopping smoking will lead to them not coping. For some people smoking is a way to relax. Smoking may be associated with positive social environments. Some people simply enjoy smoking and do not wish to stop that source of enjoyment and pleasure. Some people may deny that smoking is harmful. Stopping smoking can be extremely difficult for some people as it is an addictive behaviour.
Safe alcohol intake	Alcohol consumption is often associated with social interaction and celebration. There can be negative social pressures to consume alcohol and it can be difficult for individuals to go against that social pressure. In some cultures, this will particularly be so with men. Not consuming alcohol may be seen by some as less masculine. Peer pressure can be very powerful and difficult to resist. This is often the case with adolescents and young adults. Some people will be physically alcohol dependent and will require additional and specialist support. Alcohol is frequently used to help people relax and they may have reached a stage where they believe they cannot relax without it. Lack of awareness about safe levels of alcohol consumption. Lack of understanding about units of alcohol. Many people are unaware that their intake of alcohol is above the safe level. They may consume a lot less alcohol than people around them and therefore believe that their intake is acceptable.

Possible challenges when working with healthcare professionals

There also may be barriers when working with groups of healthcare professionals. Many work environments are extremely pressured and the expectations that staff members will take further responsibility for promoting specific types of behaviour change may not be well received.

Some individuals may also have personal agendas in relation to certain lifestyle changes. For example, trying to encourage a healthcare professional to promote smoking cessation to their patients when they smoke themselves may be difficult. Similarly, there can be challenges in the area of weight management as the messages received can be perceived as personal by participants who struggle to manage their own weight. The communication skills and empathy of the facilitator are extremely important in these situations.

Alternatively, participants may not always be empathic in relation to their patients and service users. This again needs careful handling in the group education session. An example of this type of situation is described in Box 2.1.

This chapter has discussed the area of behaviour change and how that may be supported in the group education setting. Behaviour change needs to be considered from the planning stages, in teaching methods, in relation to behaviour change interventions and techniques and also how behaviour

---

Box 2.1 Example of barrier with a healthcare professional

The group education session was designed to support healthcare professionals to promote physical activity.

Participant A was extremely fit, single, with no dependents and on a reasonable income suggested that most barriers to physical activity were simply excuses and that anyone could find time to go to the gym three times a week if they could be bothered to.

Participant B became extremely angry and distressed by this comment. She was a single parent of a child who had severe Attention Deficit Hyperactivity Disorder (ADHD) and was physically violent. She was struggling financially. She knew she should be more physically active and would have loved to have been able to get to the gym regularly but was unable to find someone willing to look after her child. She could not afford to pay for the childcare or a gym membership.

The skills of the facilitator are extremely important in situations like this. The facilitator needed to acknowledge the challenges that participant B was facing at the same time as suggesting that participant A considered that other people's situations may be more challenging than their own.

change can be measured in the evaluation. Recognizing the barriers that individual participants face and demonstrating empathy for those whilst working with participants to problem solve and plan actions is challenging but can also increase the effectiveness of our group education.

References

Ajzen I (1991). The theory of planned behaviour. *Organ Behav Hum Dec Processes* 50: 179–211.
Becker MH (Ed) (1974). *The Health Belief Model and Personal Health Behaviour.* New Jersey: Slack, Thorofare.
Bodenheimer T and Handley MA (2009). Goal-setting for behavior change in primary care: An exploration and status report. *Patient Educ Couns* 76: 174–180.
Cullen KW, Baranowski T and Smith SP (2001). Using goal setting as a strategy for dietary behavior change. *J Am Diet Assoc* 101: 562–566.
Davidson KW, Goldstein M, Kaplan RM, Kaufman PG, Knatterud GL et al. (2003). Evidence-based behavioural medicine: What is it and how do we achieve it? *Ann Behav Med* 26(3): 161–171. Available from: DOI: 10.1207/S15324796ABM2603_01 [Accessed November 2015].
Locke EA and Latham GP (2006). New directions in goal-setting theory. *Curr Dir Psychol Sci* 15(5): 265–268. Available from: DOI: 10.1111/j.1467–8721.2006.00449.x [Accessed November 2015].
Michie S, van Stralen MM and West R (2011). The behaviour change wheel: A new method for characterising and designing behaviour change interventions. *Implementation Science* 6: 42.
Michie S, Richardson M, Johnston M, Abraham C, Francis J et al. (2013). The Behaviour Change Technique Taxonomy (v1) of 93 hierarchically clustered techniques: building an international consensus for the reporting of behaviour change interventions. *Ann Behav Med* 46: 81–95.
Michie S, West R, Campbell R, Brown J and Gainforth H (2014a). *ABC of Behaviour Change Theories: An Essential Resource for Researchers, Policy Makers and Practitioners.* Croydon, UK: Silverback Publishing.
Michie S, Atkins L and West R (2014b). *The Behaviour Change Wheel: A Guide to Designing Interventions.* Croydon, UK: Silverback Publishing. Available from: www.behaviourchangewheel.com/ [Accessed May 2016].
Miller CH and Bauman J (2014). Goal setting: an integral component of effective diabetes care. *Curr Diab Rep* 14: 509.
National Institute for Health and Care Excellence (NICE) (2007). *Public Health Programme Guidance No. 6, Behaviour Change: The Principles for Effective Interventions.* London: National Institute for Health and Care Excellence.
National Institute of Health and Care Excellence (NICE) (2012). Clinical Guidance 138, *Patient Experience in Adult NHS Services: Improving the Experience of Care for People Using Adult NHS Services.* London: National Institute for Health and Care Excellence.

National Institute of Health and Care Excellence (NICE) (2014). *Public Health Guidance No. 49, Behaviour Change: Individual Approaches.* London: National Institute of Health and Care Excellence.

Parker RM, Ratzan SC and Lurie N (2003). Health literacy: A policy challenge for advancing high-quality health care. *Health Affair* 22: 147–153.

Pearson D and Grace C (2012). *Weight Management: A Practitioner's Guide.* Chichester, UK: Wiley-Blackwell.

Prochaska JO and DiClemente CC (1982). Transtheoretical therapy: Towards a more integrative model of change. *Psychotherapy: Theory, Research and Practice* 19(3): 276–288.

Reyes NR, Oliver TL, Klotz AA, Lagrotte CA, Vander Veur SS *et al.* (2012). Similarities and differences between weight loss maintainers and regainers: a qualitative analysis. *J Acad Nutr Diet* 112(4): 499–505. Available from: DOI: 10.1016/j.jand.2011.11.014 [Accessed November 2015].

Sarafino EP and Smith TW (2014). *Health Psychology: Biopsychosocial Interactions,* 6th Edn. Chichester, UK: John Wiley & Sons, Ltd.

Further reading

Corcoran N (2011). *Working on Health Communication.* London: Sage Publications.

Corcoran N (ed.) (2013). *Communicating Health: Strategies for Health Promotion,* 2nd Edn. London: Sage Publications.

UCL Centre for Behaviour Change [Online]. Available from: www.ucl.ac.uk/behaviour-change [Accessed May 2016].

World Health Organisation (2015). Obesity and overweight. Fact sheet No 311 [Online]. Available from www.who.int/mediacentre/factsheets/fs311/en/ [Accessed May 2016].

Chapter 3 **What makes a good facilitator?**

Amanda Avery

Group facilitators have a key role to play in the success of a group education programme. They are the 'change agent'. Group facilitators need both the theoretical knowledge and the ability to share this knowledge with different audiences in order to achieve the best outcomes for the target group. In fact, facilitation is the art, not of putting ideas into people's heads, but of drawing ideas out. Facilitators need to have a good understanding of how people learn and the underpinning learning theories; behavioural, cognitive, humanistic, social and situational (as discussed in Chapter 2). Facilitators need to encourage individual members of a group to reflect on how their behaviours influence their health and well-being.

'Facilitation is a technique by which one person makes things easier for others'. (Kitson *et al.*, 1998).

Facilitating an effective support group begins with a commitment to three basic assumptions:
1 that each member can make a contribution to the group
2 that each member is in control of their own needs and what will work best for them
3 that communications will be open and honest to promote positive group experiences.

How to Facilitate Lifestyle Change: Applying Group Education in Healthcare, First Edition.
Amanda Avery, Kirsten Whitehead and Vanessa Halliday.
© 2017 John Wiley & Sons, Ltd. Published 2017 by John Wiley & Sons, Ltd.

3.1 The good facilitator

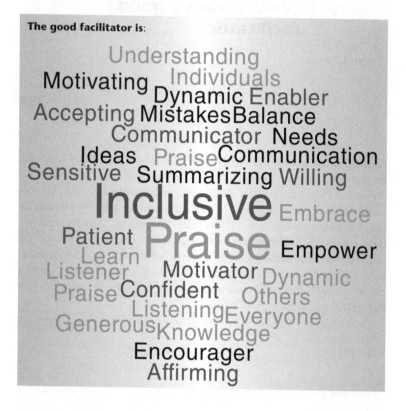

The good facilitator is:

Understanding
Motivating Individuals
Dynamic Enabler
Accepting Mistakes Balance
Communicator Needs
Ideas Praise Communication
Sensitive Summarizing Willing
Inclusive Embrace
Patient Praise Empower
Learn
Listener Motivator Dynamic
Praise Confident Others
Listening Everyone
Generous Knowledge
Encourager
Affirming

Group facilitators are confident through training, support and having the appropriate personal qualities. Key **attributes** include;

- Awareness of group behaviours – it is useful to understand how people behave in groups and to use this knowledge wisely. The Tuckman model, which looks at the different stages of group formation, is explored in more detail later in this chapter.
- Are committed to the self-care process.
- Are able to enthusiastically work towards the group's goals – they need to see themselves as part of a team and are emotionally and physically committed to the team's success. They actively and creatively look for ways to give members the opportunity to participate in the process of setting and contributing to the group's goals.
- Are able to control their own personal views – they should not have their own agenda and they need to be able to separate their own personal needs from those of the group members.

- Have the ability to initiate activity – whilst the aim is to develop shared responsibility and ownership of the group, there will be times when the facilitator will need to initiate direction on behalf of the rest of the group.
- Are comfortable with expressed emotions, including tension and conflict – good communication skills are essential to enable the facilitator to best cope with any emotions that may emerge from within the group.
- Emphasize the positive aspects of the group – an effective facilitator puts a greater emphasis on the more positive aspects such as education, learning successful coping strategies and benefitting from the support of others who genuinely understand the situation. The negatives associated with coping with the demands and consequences of a chronic condition should not be the focus.
- Encourages members to identify behavioural strategies for themselves – the effective facilitator does not directly tell people what to do but, instead, provides the nurturing environment whereby they are able to come up with their own personal solutions.
- Are 100% committed to the welfare of the group and all its members – there is something about going the extra mile to ensure that the given audience is best supported even if it requires providing additional support outside of the group.

The use of **social media** can be an effective way of providing this additional support. A good facilitator will focus on building a sense of community, group cohesiveness and consensus decision making within the group.

- Value and respect each member as an individual – whilst the focus is upon the group they do not lose sight of the individual. Members need to be seen as valued equals and each as a potential teacher, having a reservoir of knowledge and experience from which others may benefit (www.wichita.edu/ccsr).

TOP TIPS: KEY SKILLS OF A GOOD FACILITATOR INCLUDE:

- Being well prepared whilst remaining flexible
- Thinking and acting creatively using a variety of techniques, methods and activities
- Drawing energy from outside themselves rather than from within
- Thinking positively
- The ability to deal with sensitive issues and manage people's feelings
- Encouraging both humour and respect
- Negotiating with and influencing others
- The ability to keep to time without being driven by it
- The ability to gain the respect and trust of the group members
- Enthusiastic and passionate about the subject.

Put simply, the role of the facilitator is:
- Questioning
- Guiding
- Supporting
- Encouraging
- Giving feedback.

They are the 'guide on the side'. More like a coach than a manager.

They are not:
- Directing
- Telling
- Imposing
- Judgemental.

They are not the 'sage on the stage'.

The facilitator's role is to draw out knowledge and ideas from different members of a group and to help them learn from each other and yet think and act together. Facilitation is about **empowering** others (Clarke, Blackman and Carter, 2004). It can be incredibly difficult for some healthcare workers to have all the answers but not to enforce them and to let go of the control and to facilitate sharing of ideas, which may not be their own.

3.2 Communication skills for a group facilitator

Good communication skills are essential for a group facilitator. This really starts as soon as group participants arrive for a group education session. The welcome that participants receive can influence the remainder of the session. It is the opportunity for the facilitator to build rapport with them and an opportunity that should not be missed. Participants need to feel welcomed, they may need help to relax and feel at ease, they need to feel it is a supportive environment. It is really easy to underestimate the importance of the initial impression that a participant gets when they arrive for a group education session. Here are a few key points of particular relevance to the beginning of the session:

- Smile and be friendly! Give good eye contact.
- Be welcoming. You can thank people for coming or tell them that it is good to have them at the session.
- Introduce yourself and your role so the participant knows exactly who you are. It may not be obvious to them when they arrive.
- Check the name of the participant, including what they would actually like to be called. Names are important.
- Check that the individual is in the right place. Tell them about the group so that you can check that they are meant to be there. People can feel very

foolish if they are in the wrong place. You may have a list of participants that you are expecting and asking people to sign in can soon identify if someone is not expected.

- Make sure the participants know where to sit. It may be that they are free to sit anywhere but they may not know that.
- Wherever possible, check that participants are comfortable. This may include adjusting the room temperature or moving chairs to ensure people can see what they need to see.
- You may wish to direct people to a drink or let them know some of the housekeeping issues, such as where the toilets are if they need them. It is much easier for people to have this explained to them than having to ask. Sometimes people don't know if there is time to do this prior to the session starting. Clear messages can be really helpful.
- Try to include some small talk, or safe talk. For example, commenting about the weather is always a safe topic. You could ask about the journey that the participant has had or whether they found the location easily or not. This gives you an opportunity to find out if someone has had a bad experience. Being given an opportunity to talk about that can help the participant to put it behind them and better focus on the group session. Make sure you don't use the same phrase or question for each participant as they arrive. Other participants may observe this and it may seem more like a task that you need to tick off your list rather than genuine interest in the individual. Individualize the small talk if you can.
- Remember that participants may be quite anxious about the group session. A good facilitator will be mindful of this and ensure that participants are welcomed and everything that is possible is done to make them feel more at ease.
- Be mindful of your non-verbal communication. If you are running late or disorganized it is easy to communicate that to the participants. They may get the impression that you don't have time for them or that you are unprofessional. Try to avoid keeping people waiting.
- Giving a clear outline of the time frame for the group session can be very helpful. People may be anxious about leaving on time or have misunderstood the time frame for the group. Clarifying this at the beginning can avoid problems later in the session, particularly if people need to leave very promptly.
- Be mindful of your reaction if somebody is late. They still need to be welcomed. They still need to know where to sit or what expectations there are. If the rest of the group have already started an activity, then that activity will have to be explained to the latecomer. It is easy for an unguarded expression to suggest to the participant that their late arrival is unacceptable or has inconvenienced you as facilitator. Try to make your welcome as genuine and helpful as it was for those who arrived on time.

Establishing rapport

The need to establish rapport with patients is clearly defined in many policy documents (Department of Health, 2010; NICE, 2012) but it is equally important whoever the participants are. Rapport has been defined as 'a close and harmonious relationship in which the people or groups concerned understand each other's feelings or ideas and communicate well' (*Oxford English Dictionary* online). This clearly is important for effective group education and it is the group facilitator's responsibility to take the first steps to developing rapport. Good communication skills need to continue throughout the education session. It is easy to lose rapport if you fail to engage appropriately with group participants. Your active listening skills will be vitally important as building and maintaining rapport can be achieved by demonstrating respect, acceptance and empathy, ensuring you avoid being judgemental in any way.

It is important to observe your group throughout the session. If you have developed and maintained rapport with group participants they should be looking relaxed, they may be communicating with each other and with you, they will be asking appropriate questions and be willing to talk and contribute to the session.

Active listening skills

Active listening skills are well recognized as being important in one-to-one consultations. However, they are equally important in group education sessions. How we respond to group members will affect how the session progresses.

Here are some of the skills that you might want to consider:

- Minimal encouragers. These are small phrases that encourage participants to keep talking and are a good way of conveying that you are listening, for example, 'uh huh', 'go on', 'yes', 'mm', 'so' and 'I see'. One of the important aspects about these phrases is that they are neutral, which avoids you conveying agreement or disagreement or judgement. It is best to avoid words such as 'okay' or 'right', which can convey agreement with what is being said rather than active listening. There will be comments that participants make that the facilitator may not wish to convey agreement with.
- Verbal following. This is repeating a short sentence, phrase or word that the participant has just used. This is usually done quietly and at a lower tone, which conveys listening but should not interrupt what the participant is saying.
- Paraphrasing. When a participant has been talking the facilitator can restate what is the participant has said but in their own words rather than the participant's words. This conveys that the facilitator has not just heard the words that have been said but has understood them. In a group scenario

this can be really important to ensure that other participants have also understood what has been said. It is also particularly useful when a quietly spoken participant is facing the facilitator but other participants may not have heard what has been said. The facilitator should check that their paraphrase was accurate by using a short question such as 'Is that right?'

- Reflection of feelings. It is not unusual for group participants to convey emotional reactions or feelings during an education session. How the facilitator responds to this is extremely important. Ignoring the feelings expressed will have a negative impact on the participants who will feel that their feelings are not being considered important or valid. It can be very hurtful when someone has expressed emotion but others act as if it hasn't happened. Facilitators should convey that they are trying to understand participant's emotions by verbally reflecting what they think participant is expressing. For example, 'it sounds as if this has been a very difficult time for you' or 'this diagnosis has been quite a shock for you'. Some facilitators may be anxious about acknowledging emotional reactions within a group setting but ignoring feelings does not make them go away. Most participants will not expect the facilitator to have a solution for their situation or emotion but if the facilitator acknowledges that they have heard and understood the emotions they are demonstrating empathy. This helps to maintain rapport and makes the participant feel cared for. If the participant is extremely emotional it may be that the facilitator needs to offer them an opportunity to take some time out or talk to them at the end of the session. Supporting the rest of the group to undertake an activity and then talking to that individual on a one-to-one may be helpful way forward.

Table 3.1 illustrates some examples commonly seen in practice. In most cases acknowledging the emotion involved is going to be a helpful and appropriate response.

- **Questions**. It is highly likely that the facilitator will need to ask questions during the group education session. In order to invite group discussion, they may need to be open questions. In some cases, the facilitator may have a list of questions on a presentation or flip chart so that the participants can work through these in small groups. It is best to avoid multiple questions without giving time for participants to respond, questions that are asking more than one thing in the same sentence or unnecessarily complicated questions. It is extremely important to use everyday language and to keep questions clear. Questions also need to be focussed so that the discussion does not go into areas that are not relevant to the aim and learning outcomes of the session. Questions that are used in a motivational interviewing style can also work well in the group setting. See next for more about motivational interviewing in the group setting.

Table 3.1 Some common emotional situations in group education.

Emotion	Examples	Possible facilitator response
Distress	Participant realizes that they are more overweight than they thought they were.	• Acknowledge that this is a distressing situation. • It may help the participant to know that their situation is very common and many people do not realize this. • Emphasize that the group education is designed to provide information and support to help them start tackling their weight (assuming that it will do so). • Subtly monitor how the participant is during the session and offer to speak with them during a break or at the end. • Offer support or referral to another appropriate service if necessary and appropriate.
	The overall aim seems an impossible target	• Reinforce that when it comes to setting goals these will be individual and work around what that participant feels is realistic in their life. • Break the aim down into smaller more manageable goals. One step at a time!
Frustration	The participant may have tried to change their lifestyle before, without success	• Many people have repeatedly tried to change their lifestyle and the facilitator should positively affirm their previous efforts and acknowledge that it is not always easy. • It may be helpful to explore what they have tried before, what worked well (even if it was temporary) and what did not work for them and why. This can lead to a clearer idea of what is likely to work in the future. • Facilitating a group discussion can lead to other participants sharing their challenges and how they overcame them. This can be very supportive.

(Continued)

Table 3.1 (Continued)

Emotion	Examples	Possible facilitator response
	The participant may have another factor which negatively impacts on their ability to change their lifestyle, e.g. a disability or illness that limits their physical activity	• Acknowledge the difficulties. • Focus on what that person can do rather than on what they can't. • Be realistic.
Anger	Some participants may feel they should have known about the impact that their lifestyle was having before now. Why has no-one ever told me about this before?	• Acknowledge their anger about the situation. • Acknowledge that it would have been better to know earlier (without getting involved in blaming anyone for not having told them specifically). • Focus on the benefits of change now and how they can move forwards.
	How have I been fooled by misinformation? The participant may be feeling foolish or stupid.	• Acknowledge their anger about the situation • Acknowledge that there is a lot of information available which is not based on scientific evidence and that much of it is believed widely. This should help them feel less stupid for having believed what they had heard. • Direct them to appropriate information sources to help them avoid being in a similar situation again.
Encouraged	Participants may feel empowered by the group education and support.	• Affirm the positive emotional situation. • Ensure that participants remain realistic about the goals that they are setting. When people feel very enthusiastic they sometimes set goals that are too challenging. This can then lead to discouragement if they fail to achieve.

- **Summarizing**. A summary pulls together part or all of a conversation, focussing on key points. It may include both content and emotions. Facilitators can use summaries at various points in a group education session. For example, when a participant has given a long and complicated response to a question, to pull together key points from a group discussion prior to moving on to another subject, to check participants' understanding of what has been said, and at the end to recap on the content of the session. If there are activities for participants to complete before the next session, it can be helpful to summarize those as a reminder. Good summaries can really help keep the focus within an education session, particularly if participants are prone to going of the subject. It can be helpful to signpost to participants that you are going to summarize, for example 'Could I just summarize where we've got to so far?' It may be that you can get participants to summarize as a way of checking their understanding and what they think the key points of the session have been. The facilitator can then fill in any gaps or correct any misunderstanding that has been conveyed.
- All of these skills can be used to good effect in group education sessions. They are important for developing and maintaining rapport, keeping focus and checking understanding.

Motivational interviewing in the group setting

Motivational interviewing aims to enhance self-efficacy and personal control for behaviour change. It uses an interactive, empathetic listening style to increase motivation and confidence by a focussed approach. Motivational interviewing helps people to explore and resolve ambivalence (Miller and Rollnick, 2002). The main goals of motivational interviewing are to engage people and to encourage '**change talk**': it is much better to get the individual to come up with the changes they need to make and to encourage 'group change talk' with sharing of ideas. The group member needs to resolve his or her own ambivalence to change.

Group facilitators could consider some of the following types of questions to encourage the group members to think about their behaviours:

- How do you feel about changing your lifestyle behaviours (eating, exercising, smoking, drinking etc.)?
- How would you like your health to be different?
- How ready do you feel to change your lifestyle behaviours?
- How is your current weight affecting your life?
- What kind of things have you done in the past to change your lifestyle/behaviours? Are there things that you have found helpful?
- What strategies have worked for you in the past?

- What would make you more confident about making changes?
- What barriers might get in the way of you being able to make lifestyle changes?
- What are your hopes for the future if you are able to become healthier?
- What do you think might happen if you don't make any lifestyle changes?

The facilitator might discuss with the group what they perceive to be the short-term and long-term benefits and drawbacks of making healthy changes: they could, as a group, list five short-term benefits, five long-term benefits and compare these with the respective costs (www. motivationalinterviewing.org).

Emotional intelligence

Emotional intelligence embraces and draws from numerous other branches of behavioural, emotional and communication theories but with a real focus on empathy. Emotional intelligence is defined as the ability to monitor one's own and other people's emotions, to discriminate between different emotions and label them appropriately and to use emotional information to guide thinking and behaviour (Goleman, 1995). Emotions include personal values, beliefs, attitudes and habits, which will have been embedded from an early age, besides the more basic human emotional needs. Some emotions can be based on long-term memories and serve as a protective reaction to a certain situation. For example, chocolate or other confectionary may have been given to a child when they were upset to try and cheer them up and make them feel less sad about a distressing situation.

Working with emotions and facilitating with emotional intelligence is likely to be a more persuasive model to employ when facilitating behaviour change. A very easy way of achieving this is by asking members of the group about how they feel about different situations and challenges that they might be facing. With confidence asking about feelings can be a useful asset to have at different time-points and can be a useful form of evaluation.

We all essentially have two minds, one that thinks and one that feels. Influencing the thinking mind may lead to changes in knowledge and skills but influencing the emotional mind and people's feelings is more likely to lead to changes in attitude and habits. In the words of Aristotle, 'educating the mind without educating the heart is no education at all'.

A good example is the use of medication to manage certain lifestyle conditions without any additional support to change how one was feeling and then being taken off the medication. Without the medication, the person is going to be as vulnerable to relapse as they were before they took the medication. The medication alone is not going to change attitudes and habits that have been deeply embedded.

Importance of non-verbal communication

Being a good communicator requires more than just good verbal skills; often what you say is less important than how you say it or other non-verbal signals such as gestures you make, tone of voice or how much eye contact you make. In order to gain the trust and attention of the group, the facilitator needs to be aware of their body language and also to be aware and respond to the non-verbal cues from members of the group.

If the facilitator wants to have an attentive group, they in need to be attentive, at all times, to the needs of the group.

We all know that laughter and humour can be natural antidotes to life's difficulties. They can help lighten the burden and help keep things in perspective. In the group environment, the facilitator can use warmth, humour and laughter with good effect to help manage tensions. With experience, humour can be used to help discuss issues that may otherwise be difficult to express but it is important that this is done in a non-stigmatizing way, as discussed later.

A smile is going to make people feel much more welcomed and feeling good about themselves compared to a facilitator who looks as if they do not want to be there.

3.3 How do effective groups form?

The facilitator also needs a good understanding of how groups come together and how they may behave at each of the key stages. The Tuckman model (Tuckman, 1965 and cited by many others), suggests that there are five stages that groups go through; from forming to storming, to norming, to performing and then to adjourning. These stages might occur during a single group session or across a series of group sessions. If only a single group session is offered, then the duration of each of the stages is going to be quite brief but still remain important to acknowledge.

In the **forming stage**, following a warm welcome, group members are introduced. They may indicate how they came to be at the group and their hopes and fears of being part of the group. Members may explore the boundaries of acceptable group behaviour, particularly children. The forming is a stage of transition from individual to member status and of assessing the facilitator's guidance both formally and informally.

Forming may include some of these feelings and behaviours, which will differ between individuals and from group to group:
- Some excitement, anticipation and optimism.
- Pride in being chosen or referred to the group.
- A tentative attachment to the 'team'.

- Some suspicion and anxiety about the programme.
- Determining acceptable group behaviour.
- Defining the tasks and how they will be accomplished.
- Deciding what information needs to be gathered.
- Abstract discussions of the concepts and issues with difficulty identifying relevant problems.
- Perhaps some impatience.

Given there is so much going on to distract members' attention in this forming stage, the group will achieve little, if anything, towards meeting the programmes aim and objectives. This is perfectly normal and needs to be accepted as an important element of the process. A good facilitator is willing to spend time in building relationships rather than always being task orientated. Hopes and fears need to be addressed as part of the introductions.

Storming

The group's transition from the forming to a more productive stage is called the **storming phase**. During this next stage, all members can still have their own ideas as to how the group should work with some personal agendas being difficult to manage. Storming is probably the most difficult stage for the group as they begin to realize that the tasks ahead are different and more difficult than they had thought. Individuals may become impatient about the lack of progress; they may argue about just what actions the group should be taking. They may try to rely on their own personal and professional experiences and resist collaboration with most of the other group members.

Storming includes these feelings and behaviours:

- Establishing unrealistic goals.
- Resisting the tasks.
- Resisting ideas suggested by other members.
- Arguing among members even when they agree on the real issues.
- Defensiveness, competition and choosing sides.
- Fluctuations in attitude about the team and the programme's chance of success.
- Questioning the wisdom of those who developed and selected the programme and referred the other members.
- Disunity, increased tension and jealousy.

The listed feelings and behaviours could mean that group members have little energy to spend on progressing towards the group's goal(s), but at least they are beginning to understand one another. This stage sometimes takes three or four meetings before arriving at the norming phase, but can be shorter if the majority of members have incentives that they identify with. But it is definitely the most difficult phase for the group facilitator to manage.

Norming

The **norming phase** occurs when members reach a consensus on how the group is going to work and there is some united focus. Everyone wants to share this newly found focus. Enthusiasm is high and the group is ambitious to go beyond the original scope of the programme. During this stage, emotional conflict is reduced as members reconcile competing loyalties and responsibilities. They accept the group, ground rules, their roles in the group and the individuality of fellow members.

Norming includes these feelings and behaviours:

- An ability to both express and receive criticism constructively.
- A sense of team cohesion, spirit and goals.
- Acceptance of membership in the 'team'.
- More friendliness, confiding in each other and sharing of personal problems.
- An attempt to achieve harmony by avoiding conflict.
- Accepting and maintaining ground rules and boundaries.

As group members begin to share their personal problems and forget their differences, they now have more time and energy to spend on the programme of self-care and of coming up with some solutions themselves.

Performing

The stage occurs when the group and 'team' members have settled their relationships and expectations. They can begin **performing** by diagnosing, coming up with solutions and solving problems, and choosing and implementing changes. At last group members have discovered and accepted each other's strengths and weakness, and learned how they can have an active and productive role.

Performing includes these feelings and behaviours:

- Close attachment to the team.
- Members have insights into personal and group processes, and better understanding of each other's strengths and weakness.
- Ability to prevent or work through group problems.
- Constructive self-change.

The group is now an effective, cohesive unit. You can tell when the group has reached this stage because they start achieving more of the goals and desired outcomes. One of the most important attributes of a good facilitator is the ability to provide encouragement and praise for all achievements, no matter how small. Small changes achieved by each group member should be recognized. Constructive feedback acknowledges achievements but also includes communication as to how the achievements may be even greater by getting people to reflect on how they come so far and how they can go even further. The group support is very powerful in this process as they generate solutions, share tips and ideas and what has worked for them. Generally, a more solution-focussed approach works better than a problem-based approach. Barriers to change need to be acknowledged but understanding the cause of a problem is not necessarily going to help resolve it and indeed an over-focus on the barriers can sometimes get in the way of change.

Adjourning

This stage of the group forming and working together process is often over-looked and yet it is so important. When the group finally completes that last meeting, there can be a bittersweet sense of achievement coupled with the reluctance to say good-bye and let go. Many relationships formed within a group continue long after the group disbands and these relationships can help to ensure that lifestyle changes achieved are maintained. Some informal self-help groups may be established, which is a desirable outcome, so that the peer support and self-management can continue. There is an opportunity to signpost to additional support and other services. The good facilitator will be aware of what other activities are happening locally and have resources to give out with the contact details for the various activities.

At the final group meeting it is important to celebrate the successful achievements of every group member. It could be made into a special meeting where something slightly different happens, for example there could be some food and drink offered (healthy choices) and certificates handed out by a local person of importance.

Table 3.2 provides an overall summary of this process.

There could potentially be some advantages of having a fluid membership where new members join at different time-points and members stay as part of the group for as long as they feel they are personally deriving a benefit. In this scenario the different stages may not be so obvious, and some of the conflict in the storming stage avoided and the adjourning not be so obvious with people being able to leave the group at their own choice. Some people may benefit from accessing group support for far longer than just a few sessions.

3.4 How do different people behave in groups?

Understanding how individuals react and behave in group settings can further enable the facilitator to provide the appropriate level of support. People tend to behave in one or two of eight possible roles, as identified by Belbin (1981). These roles include **implementer, coordinator, shaper, innovator, resource investigator, monitors evaluator, team worker** and **completer**, the role

Table 3.2 Summary of how effective groups form and the role the facilitator plays.

Stage	Examples of Facilitator Behaviour
Forming	Welcoming Encouraging/motivating Establishing personal incentives Encouraging 'getting to know you' activities and ice-breakers Establishing ground-rules Clarifying any uncertainties
Storming	Some protection of individuals if needed Feedback to assist in formation of team goals Praise for constructive team behaviour Questions about aims, outcomes
Norming	Encouraging a list of solutions Challenging, encouraging higher performance Constructive feedback on performance and process, including any weaknesses
Performing	Very little! Some praise and feedback Challenging to do 'even better' Persuasive communication
Adjourning	Evaluation/reflections Celebration Congratulation Discussion of 'what next' and how to maintain the changes achieved Signposting

names being reasonably self-explanatory. The most effective group will include members with each of these defined characteristics and not too many of any one type but of course we are not always in charge of the group membership. It is good to have a number of team workers, a couple of resource investigators, but we also need people who have innovative ideas and others who take a lead, monitor progress and get things completed. The larger the group, the more likely each of these roles will be represented.

The clever facilitator will identify these characteristics in people within the group as soon as possible and will endeavour to ensure that the strengths of each of these attributes is used effectively.

Additional skills are required to support people from disadvantaged backgrounds who may have very low incomes and/or low educational attainment with limited literacy skills. Very practical sessions are going to be more valuable to this audience and the aim should be to empower rather than disempower and to recognize that it might be more difficult for some people to make changes compared to others. In these circumstances it is really important to give praise for any small changes in the right direction.

The same applies for people with a low self-esteem, who for many reasons may have little confidence in their own ability and who also will benefit from additional praise.

The importance of using non-stigmatizing communication

All individual members of a group are potentially quite vulnerable, again for many different reasons. It is well recognized that if someone has a chronic long-term condition they are up to more than 20% more likely to suffer from depression (Moussavi *et al.*, 2007). When a person is labelled or marked by their illness, then they are seen as part of a stereotyped group. Negative attitudes create prejudice which can lead to negative actions and discrimination. Stigma brings experiences and feelings of shame, blame, hopelessness, distress and a reluctance to seek and/or accept necessary help. so it is vitally important that group facilitators do not use stigmatizing language and resources.

'Anti-fat attitude', 'weight stigma', 'weight bias' and 'anti-fat prejudice' are terms referred to in the literature that describe a negative attitude (dislike of), belief about (stereotype) or behaviour against (discrimination) people perceived as being fat (Danielsdottir *et al.*, 2010).

There is a large body of evidence that suggests overweight or obese people are particularly stigmatized and that healthcare practitioners can be a source of this stigma. Some healthcare practitioners may blame people for having developed their condition. We all need to question whether we are the source of any negative attitudes, prejudice or discrimination as this can be harmful to an individual's well-being, including to their self-esteem.

TOP TIPS: HOW TO AVOID STIGMATIZING LANGUAGE

- Do not label people: a person has diabetes, they are not diabetic.
- Do not stereotype people either through one's language or through the resources and images used.
- Suggest that someone's condition implies negative assumptions about their character, intelligence or abilities.
- Do not be seen to judge people.
  Instead, treat all group members, whatever their condition, with respect and dignity, as you would anyone else.

As mentioned previously, it is particularly overweight and obese people where stigma is experienced. Instead of saying 'because you are obese your health will suffer', change this for 'if you are able to lose some weight, your health will benefit'. You are still being accurate and not dodging the truth. In fact, people generally do not like being called obese; it is a medical term perhaps best used only for research purposes. Also, do not use fat jokes or humour and think about images used in resources.

The Uconn Rudd Center for Food Policy and Obesity has an excellent toolkit for health professionals to use to guide their communications with this vulnerable and often very sensitive population group (www.uconnruddcenter.org).

The facilitator as a role model

It can be questioned as to whether the facilitator should also be seen as a role model where their behavioural decisions can be seen as an example of success that can be desirable to and emulated by the group members. For example, should a person facilitating a weight management group be a person who has successfully managed to lose weight themselves? Should the person who is encouraging an increase in activity levels successfully manage to incorporate activity in their busy lives? Should the person who is facilitating a smoking cessation group be a successful quitter? The concept of role models was first described many years ago (Rakestraw and Weiss, 1981) where it was proposed that individuals compare themselves with reference groups of people who occupy the social role to which the individual aspires. High achieving role models gain greater respect and provide greater motivation. Ideally, role modelling will come from both the group facilitator and other members of the group and there can be benefits from successful group members being retained so that they are supported, not only to maintain their lifestyle changes, but also to inspire others. However, if the group facilitator is struggling to manage their own weight or to stop smoking that does not mean that they cannot facilitate a weight management or stop smoking group, but ideally they should be seen to also be trying to address their lifestyle and thus improve their own health. The empathy with the group members, being honest and acknowledging that they too are benefitting from the support and sharing of ideas, can be quite powerful. This may be more acceptable if it is a lay person facilitating the group rather than a healthcare professional, particularly for behaviours like smoking.

Even if one is an excellent role model it is important to acknowledge that no one is perfect. For behaviours such as eating and food choices, even if one's weight is in the healthy range, no one eats the perfect diet all the time. It is just that the role model will have strategies in place to ensure that their weight does not increase.

3.5 And finally...

Passion and enthusiasm have been described as important attributes of the group facilitator. They are! The group experience should be fun and enjoyable with the group members wanting to come back.

References

Belbin RM (1981). *Management Teams: Why They Succeed or Fail.* Oxford: Butterworth-Heinemann.

Clarke S, Blackman R and Carter I (2004). *Facilitation Skills Workbook.* England: Tearfund.

Danielsdottir S, O'Brien KS and Ciao A (2010). Anti-fat prejudice reduction: a review of published studies. *Obe. Facts* 3: 47–58.

Department of Health (2010). *Essence of Care Benchmarks for Communication.* London: The Stationery Office Limited.

Goleman D (1995). *Emotional Intelligence; Why It Can Matter More than IQ.* Bloomsbury Publishing Plc, London.

Kitson A, Harvey G and McCormack B (1998). Enabling the implementation of evidence based practice: a conceptual framework. *Qual Health Care* 7: 149–158.

Miller WR and Rollnick S (2002). *Motivational Interviewing: Preparing People to Change Addictive Behaviour.* 2nd Edn. New York: Guilford Press.

Moussavi S, Chatterji S, Verdes E, Tandon A, Patel V and Ustun B (2007). Depression, chronic diseases and decrements to health: results from the World Health Surveys. *Lancet* 370(9590): 851–858.

National Institute for Health and Care Excellence (NICE) (2012). *Patient Experience in Adult NHS Services (CG138).* London: National Institute for Health and Care Excellence.

Oxford English Dictionary (n.d.) Website, available online at: www.oxforddictionaries. com/definition/english/rapport (accessed 7 April 2015).

Rakestraw TL and Weiss HM (1981). The interaction of social influences and task experience on goals, performance and performance satisfaction. *Organ Behav Hum Perf* 27: 326–344.

Tuckman BW (1965). Developmental sequence in small groups. *Psychol Bull* 63: 384–399.

Chapter 4 **Planning and organization**

Kirsten Whitehead

4.1 Introduction

There is a lot to consider when planning and organizing a group education session. In most cases a better planned session will be more successful. Although some facilitators may be willing and able to adapt or 'ad lib' successfully, this usually comes from having delivered many sessions previously, being extremely familiar with the current evidence base and material being delivered and having learnt from many mistakes or challenging situations in the past. Some people make it look easy! However, more often, poor planning will lead to a poorly prepared and delivered session that does not meet its aim and objectives. There are many possible negative outcomes from a poor education session including waste of healthcare resources, missed opportunity to promote health and behaviour change, participants may be reluctant to attend other educational sessions in the future and they may continue with unhealthy behaviours leading to poorer health outcomes. Unhappy participants may also share their views of the session with others and discourage their attendance. It is clear that one poor session could have much wider negative consequences and that good quality group education is essential. Although no group education is going to be perfect and meet every participant's needs on every occasion, careful planning and thorough organizational processes increase the likelihood of success.

In many situations a pack of information will be produced to enable the same group education session to be delivered repeatedly to different groups of participants but who have the same information and health needs. It is likely that such sessions may be delivered by different facilitators. This increases the likelihood of inconsistency in content and delivery and consequently inconsistency with outcomes. A well prepared education session

How to Facilitate Lifestyle Change: Applying Group Education in Healthcare, First Edition.
Amanda Avery, Kirsten Whitehead and Vanessa Halliday.

will have sufficient documentation to allow it to be delivered repeatedly and by different (suitably qualified) facilitators to a consistent and high standard.

This chapter will discuss a range of practical factors that will equip facilitators to plan, develop and deliver effective, acceptable and consistently high quality education sessions to participants. For consistency, unless otherwise stated, the chapter will assume one facilitator and one education session rather than groups of sessions and multiple facilitators.

4.2 What are the priorities for group education?

There is a need to prioritize the education sessions that are likely to lead to the greatest improvements in health outcomes. That could be by educating patients, carers, healthcare professionals or other staff involved in the care and support of patients and carers.

There are several key considerations when prioritizing that include:

- What are the policy drivers and guidance that are affecting the service being provided? This could include government policy, national guidance, for example NICE guidance, local health priorities and professional guidance. Using these along with the published literature in the subject area help provide a clear rationale to those who fund health services;

- Service specification, that is, what is the facilitator's organization or department being commissioned to deliver? If they are not being paid to deliver education on a specific subject, then the development of the education session is unlikely to be supported;

- The facilitator's role and professional boundaries, that is, are they qualified to provide this education? Do they have the required knowledge and skills? Do they need to involve another facilitator with a different knowledge base or skill set?

- Is there an area where a group education session would be a really important service development that would lead to improved patient care and increased efficiency? Developing a thoroughly evaluated pilot would provide evidence as to the effectiveness of the session and could support a bid for funding.

TOP TIP

Is the priority of your service the same as another working locally? Might the two services be able to work in partnership?

4.3 Needs assessment

Having identified a subject area that is a priority it is important to consider the specific learning needs of the participants. Increasingly in healthcare, participants' needs are being investigated to allow the development of more bespoke educational sessions and services (e.g. Gillespie *et al.*, 2015; James *et al.*, 2015). This can be undertaken by meeting with participants individually, as a group or undertaking a survey or telephone interview. Data needs to be gathered to identify participant characteristics such as current knowledge, skills, abilities, age range, gender, educational level, occupation, culture, health problem and factors that influence their lifestyle (Holli *et al.*, 2014). The need for learning is the gap between what participants already know and what they should know (Holli *et al.*, 2014). This will help clearly identify what is required and at what level, which makes the education session more likely to be effective.

4.4 Subject areas for group education

In relation to lifestyle change these will include increasing physical activity and reducing sedentary behaviour, smoking cessation, healthy eating, prevention and management of overweight and obesity, behaviour change and safe alcohol consumption. Some of these subjects might be delivered as an overview in one session or a series of education sessions might be required, depending on the needs of the target participants. For example, a healthy eating group might have a series of education sessions including how to decrease fat intake, reducing sugar or salt intake, increasing intake of fruit and vegetables and so on. It might also include very practical skills based sessions such as how to eat well on a low budget or cooking healthy family meals. Weight management groups are likely to include education around healthy eating, appropriate portion sizes, physical activity and behaviour change in line with recommendations (NICE, 2014). They should also consider the need to prevent weight regain.

In some cases, the type of education required will be clearly defined and cardiac rehabilitation is a good example of this. The British Association for Cardiovascular Prevention and Rehabilitation (BACPR) *Standards and Core Components for Cardiovascular Disease Prevention and Rehabilitation* sets out seven core standards that patients, healthcare professionals and commissioners should expect from a high quality cardiac rehabilitation programme. This includes:

1 Health behaviour change and education;
2 Lifestyle risk factor management, physical activity and exercise, diet and smoking cessation;
3 Psychosocial health;

4 Medical risk factor management;

5 Cardioprotective therapies;

6 Long-term management;

7 Audit and evaluation.

This document clearly specifies who should deliver the group education and who should attend it. These guidelines are part of the NICE Commissioning Guide (CMG40, 2013). Similarly, NICE Pathways (2015) recommend that structured patient education is made available to everyone with diabetes at diagnosis and then as needed. Where national guidance is available, it may be more likely that funding would be available to deliver such services.

4.5 Target participants

There are few of us who lead a perfect healthy lifestyle but providing group education for whole populations is not a practical proposition. However, there are many subsets of populations whose health is being badly affected (or likely to be badly affected in the future) and would benefit from changing their lifestyle to a healthier one. The populations at greatest risk are the priorities. This might include people at high risk of cardiovascular events, those with impaired glucose tolerance at high risk of developing type 2 diabetes, obese pregnant women at risk of increased complications during pregnancy and childbirth, those who already have heart disease or have had a cardiac event. It might include people with greater risk due to ethnicity or social deprivation. For example, there are recommendations to develop more bespoke education sessions for the prevention and management of obesity in those ethnic minority groups in England at greatest risk (Department of Health, 2010).

As there is such a great need for lifestyle change to improve health, it is important to ensure consistent messages and to take all opportunities to support health behaviour change. This is the ethos of Make Every Contact Count (MECC) where all organizations responsible for health, well-being, care and safety are being encouraged to train staff to take all opportunities, however brief, to promote health and well-being (East Midlands Health Trainer Hub, 2014). For this reason, there will be many group education sessions that are not direct to patients, but are to staff who can then support health behaviour change in a variety of ways.

4.6 Recruitment

Part of the needs assessment process will be identifying the best ways to access the target participants, particularly for hard to reach groups. Where are the target participants most likely to hear about, or read about, the education session?

Who is most likely to meet with target participants to share information with them? Who is responsible for receiving referrals or applications and completing the appropriate administration for the education session? All of this needs to be considered in order to ensure that a sufficient number of appropriate individuals are able to attend the session. The facilitator should be able to go into a session knowing how many participants are likely to turn up and who they are. There may need to be a cut-off date when a decision will be made if the session is viable ; that is, there are sufficient participants registered for the session to make it worthwhile delivering. In some cases, there may be more people wishing to attend than there are places in which case a waiting list will have to be created or further dates for delivering the session planned. A clear administration plan is essential.

Recruiting patient, service user and carer participants

There are a variety of commonly used ways to support recruitment of patient, service user and carer participants:

- Posters may be used in a variety of venues where target participants are likely to visit, for example health centres, Children's centres or community centres;
- Written information such as a flyer or information sheet can be left in areas such as waiting rooms or given to staff working in these areas to share with potential participants;
- Referrals can be made by staff working with the target participants. The referral criteria (Who is this education for?) and the referral process (What does the participant have to do to access the education?) will need to be clearly specified and a process of administration developed;
- Personal invitations can be made via letter to target participants, for example people may be identified from healthcare databases;
- For some target groups there may be community leaders who can encourage people to consider attending.
- Whatever method is used consideration must be given to possible language and literacy issues within the target population to ensure that the communication will be accessible.

Recruiting staff participants

Although some of the methods used could be similar to those for patients and carers, in many cases recruitment will be different for staff participants and the following are commonly used methods:

- Email via staff lists. Many organizations will have staff email lists and the session can be advertised using this. They may go to whole organizations or teams within them. Sometimes there will be a cascade system so that information goes to managers who can then choose whether to pass on to their staff or not;

- The session may be advertised on specific organizational web pages, for example, staff education and training departments may oversee all sessions provided within an organization. They may also deal with all of the administration;
- Posters may be used in communal work areas;
- Managers may identify a session that they feel is useful to all staff and may request a session is delivered in their department to get the maximum staff attendance.

Whatever the methods used, it is important to have a clear plan for recruitment from the start that relates directly to the participants you are trying to target.

TOP TIP

- Make sure you include all of the relevant information on a poster or flyer for a group education session:
  - What is the education about?
  - Who is it designed for?
  - Who is delivering the session?
  - Where will it be delivered?
  - What time will it be and how long will it last?
  - Who can people contact for more information? Name, role and telephone number or email address.
  - What do people who want to attend have to do?
- Always get someone to read the draft flyer or poster prior to producing multiple copies. It is really easy to miss key information that could negatively affect recruitment.
- Don't forget that more detailed information may be needed once participants have decided to attend.

4.7 Preparing for a group education session

In the process of identifying the target group (who?) and the subject area(s) (what?) for the group education session, then the rationale for the session will have been identified (why?). The next step is to consider the practicalities for delivering the session (where, when and how?)

Where? Settings and venues

There are several important considerations for deciding on a venue to deliver a group education session.

- Is the location accessible for the target participants? Is it on a bus/tram/rail/cycle/safe walking route? Is there parking (including for people with disabilities) for those travelling by car? Are there clear directions to the venue which people can access to make it easier for them? If people cannot easily get to a location, then this will decrease the chance that they will attend.

- Is the venue accessible and suitable for all participants? Does it have accessible toilet facilities? Is there a lift if the room being used is not on the ground floor? This is also important for the facilitator themselves who may have a significant amount of resources that they need to carry.

- Are there facilities to provide refreshments for participants or will refreshments have to be delivered or provided by the facilitator? This will impact on costs.

- Is there a reception area where participants can check in to the building or will the facilitator need to check people in themselves? A complete list of participants is likely to be required for fire regulations. It may also need to be given to building managers or reception staff prior to the session to ensure that only invited participants attend.

- Is the room being used suitable in terms of layout and furniture? Is there sufficient space for the number of participants and facilitator? Can the furniture be moved around if needed for small group activities? It is best to avoid having people seated in rows like a classroom where they may be looking at the back of another participant's head (Holli et al., 2014). Will participants all be able to see and hear the facilitator well and have eye contact with other participants? Is it comfortable and clean? Is there space for wheelchairs, push chairs or anything else that participants are likely to require? If working with obese participants, it is important to consider the need for suitably sized chairs without arms (NICE, 2014).

- Costs. Some venues may contain all the facilities the facilitator could wish for but the cost may be prohibitive. Is there sufficient resource to have the session there? What funding is available? Is there going to be any charge for participants attending the session? This is unlikely for patients or service users but is more likely for staff.

- If the session includes food preparation, then are there facilities where this can be undertaken safely? What is the maximum number of people who can use the facilities at any one time? The facilitator should check for evidence of risk assessments and health and safety policies. Are the facilities

Table 4.1 Information to collect when using a venue for a food-related education session. Source: Reproduced with permission of Nottingham Citycare.

Contact name and contact number

Where are the fire exits located?

Where are the fire extinguishers and blankets located?

Where is the fire evacuation assembly point?

Is there disabled access to the venue and kitchen?

Is a lone worker device required?

Is a first aid kit available? If so, where is it located?

Are there any restrictions on the use of the kitchen? (e.g. is it locked? Who is the key holder etc.? Will there be other groups/people using the kitchen at the same time?)

How many people can comfortably fit/work in the kitchen at one time?

Is the kitchen and venue clean and safe to use?

Are there any of the following available at the venue?
Oven, hobs, microwave, fridge, freezer, saucepans, cups, plates, dishes, cutlery, cooking utensils, washing up liquid

Is there a clean lidded bin available?

Is any of the equipment locked away? (e.g. knives, electrical items, plates?)

Are there any drink making facilities?

Other comments

---

safe? Has the facilitator successfully completed a food hygiene certificate? Has the venue been assessed for food hygiene? See Table 4.1 for a checklist of information to obtain.

- If physical activity is to be included are the facilities suitable for that? Again a risk assessment may be necessary. Adequate space, equipment and suitable flooring should be considered, as well as an appropriately trained facilitator.
- Is the room big enough? Some venues will limit the size of the group. If you are planning activities involving small-group discussion, having a room that allows for participants to move around and sit together in smaller gatherings is important. Having breakout areas or additional rooms is ideal as it means that participants will not have to compete with the discussion happening in other groups in order to be heard.

Commonly used venues include in and out-patient healthcare settings, community halls, health centres, care homes, workplaces, places of worship, schools, health clubs and supermarkets. It could also be that education sessions are delivered via the internet and other electronic media.

Whatever the venue, it is important to consider all these practical elements, as well as the psychological environment (Holli *et al.*, 2014). Are participants going to feel welcomed, supported and at ease when they arrive? Welcome signs on doors and clear directions to the room really help reduce stress.

TOP TIPS

- Visit potential venues prior to confirming or delivering group education sessions to ensure that they meet requirements.
- Prepare a checklist to support a consistent and thorough approach when assessing the appropriateness of a venue (see the example of a food-related education session in Table 4.1). This should be completed before the first session to confirm the suitability of the venue.

When?

The timing of group education sessions is important and will depend on the target participants. If working with young mothers, then timing a session during school hours would allow them to deliver children to school, come to the session and then leave in time to collect children. Older people may have access to free public transport within certain hours so starting a session at a time that means they do not have to pay for transport is advisable. Also some older people or people with disabilities may struggle to get moving early in the mornings and require a later start. For working adults trying to minimize time off work will be appreciated. Avoiding peak times for traffic congestion may also help.

Some group education sessions will be delivered at a workplace in order to access a particular group of participants. In this case, the timing will need to be negotiated with workplace managers who would need to release staff to attend. It may be possible to approach potential participants to assess their views on suitable timings, for example by using a survey. In some cases, a selection of possible dates can be suggested and using an online tool, such as a doodle poll (http://doodle.com/en_GB/), can allow you to ascertain when most people can attend.

What?

You may have an idea of what the content of the session needs to be but it is important to make this very specific by developing an overall aim for the session, specific objectives to guide what you are going to deliver and clear learning outcomes for participants. When writing an education session, your content should be designed to deliver the aim, objectives and learning outcomes.

> **TOP TIP**
>
> If possible, when planning a group education session, try to access views of potential participants on where and when will suit them best and what they want to know about.

What is an aim?

An **aim** is the result that your plans or action are intended to achieve (*Cambridge Dictionaries online*, 2015). It is a broad statement (Naidoo and Wills, 2009), for example 'The aim of this group education session is to increase participant awareness of the causes and management of overweight and obesity' or 'This group education session aims to support participants to increase their physical activity level'.

Usually a group education session will have one overall aim.

What is an objective?

Objectives are specific and precise statements of the intended outcomes that will contribute to the aim (Naidoo and Wills, 2009), that is, something specific that you plan to do or achieve (Cambridge Dictionaries online, 2015). All objectives for a session should contribute to the aim and they should guide the development of the content. Group education sessions will often have 3–4 objectives designed to ensure that the aim of the session is met. They help keep the focus and should be developed prior to starting to prepare the content of the session. They may need to be agreed with various stakeholders. It is useful to include the aim and objectives of a group education session when advertising it. Participants, particularly healthcare professionals, may decide whether to attend or not based on this information. It tells them if they are likely to learn relevant material or not.

What is a learning outcome?

Learning outcomes give a clear indication of the desired endpoint for the participant in the education session. They are usually written in the future tense, for example 'At the end of the session participants will be able to....'

There is extensive literature relating to this area. Bloom (1956) described three domains that learning outcomes should relate to. These are:
• Cognitive (relating to knowledge and intellectual skills)
• Psychomotor (physical skills)
• Affective (feelings, beliefs and attitudes).

The focus of the learning outcomes will relate to the aim of the session and the participants but it may be useful to think about whether aspects from these three domains need to be included. The words used to describe what participants should be able to do should relate to who they are and the knowledge and skill base they already have. Readers who wish for a more thorough and detailed review should consult Anderson *et al.* (2014).

Commonly learning outcomes are written to be SMART; **S**pecific, **M**easurable, **A**chievable, **R**esults focussed, **R**ealistic/**R**elevant and have a **T**ime frame. Let's look at these words more closely.

Specific: This means a precise detail, clearly defined, clear and exact (Cambridge Dictionaries online, 2015). For example,

'At the end of the session participants will be able to use food labels to identify foods that are high in salt (containing more than 1.5 g salt per 100 g).'

Here, there is a clear definition of what 'high in salt' means in relation to food labelling and therefore the facilitator can be clear that the foods that the participant identifies are truly 'high in salt'. This would be a really important learning outcome for a group of people with hypertension to support them to decrease their intake of foods 'high in salt'. This learning outcome is specific about food labels and salt content. A less specific learning outcome might suggest that 'At the end of the session participants will be able to identify foods that contain quite a lot of salt'. This is much less clear and precise as we don't know how they are going to identify these foods or what 'quite a lot' means. If participants only identified foods that they never ate, it is unlikely that this knowledge would lead to behaviour change. Perhaps even more specific would be to add … foods 'in their diet'… so that the knowledge becomes more relevant to the individual. Avoid vague verbs such as 'know', 'understand' and 'appreciate' as these are incredibly difficult to measure in a meaningful way. It is better to select verbs that describe what the participants will be able to do after the education session and learning has taken place, for example, recall, explain, write, use or demonstrate (Holli *et al.*, 2014).

Measurable: One way to achieve this is to add in some numbers, for example, 'At the end of the session, participants will be able to use food labels to identify five foods that are high in salt (containing more than 1.5 g salt per 100 g).'

In this way, the learning outcome would only be met if the participants had identified five foods high in salt and not just four or less. If the learning outcomes are not measurable it is very difficult to decide on whether the group education has met its objectives or not. Would it be successful if the participants could only identify one or two foods high in salt? Would that be enough to change their average salt intake and decrease their blood pressure? It is very unlikely.

It is important to be realistic about what can be measured. Often that relates to changes in knowledge (foods high in salt) or skills (how to interpret food labels) rather than behaviour change (buying and consuming lower salt foods). In effect, education sessions are often designed to change knowledge and skills with the hope (aim) that this will give participants tools to support behaviour change and that they will then implement change. Facilitators are often measuring the impact of the session (change in knowledge and skills) rather than the longer term outcome (decrease in blood pressure) that they hope will be the long term result. Actually measuring behaviour change may require a long term approach, a follow up with participants and a variety of tools. What can be measured will vary and in some cases an important health goal such as smoking cessation, increased physical fitness or weight loss can (and should) be measured. This may be measuring the impact of more than an education session or series of sessions. The resources required must be considered when deciding what to measure. This will be discussed further in Chapter 7.

Achievable or attainable: Learning outcomes have to be achievable from the session that is being delivered. Participants will only be able to use food labels to identify five foods that are high in salt if the content of the education session tells them what 'high in salt' means and how to use food labels to access that information. If the learning outcome was, 'At the end of the session, participants will be able to plan a week's menu containing no more than 6 g of salt every day' but they have only been told that the recommendation is for no more than 6 g salt a day and how to read a food label, it is unlikely that most people would be able to meet the learning outcome. There is a massive gap between what is taught and the expected outcome and that is not achievable. Often learning outcomes are written as aspirations rather than being achievable and therefore they will not be met within the education session. Learning often continues beyond the education session itself and measuring longer-term outcomes captures this.

Results focussed, relevant and realistic: What results are required from this education session? They need to be realistic and relevant for the participants. A realistic learning outcome needs to be sensible, practical and consider the ability of the participants and the resources available.

What might be realistic in the ideal world may not be remotely realistic in a limited resource situation. Taking a group of people with limited cooking skills and suggesting that they would be able to train to be chefs at the end of the session would be a very unrealistic learning outcome. Understanding the group participants prior to the session will help to prepare realistic learning outcomes. Similarly, knowledge about participants will also help to ensure that learning outcomes are relevant. The aim and learning outcomes need to be focussed on the need of the participants. What is most important and relevant to them and their needs?

Timescale: This is important and is often written as 'At the end of the session...', but that is not always going to be appropriate. You cannot expect that a participant will increase their physical activity by 1000 steps per day at the end of the session. They may, however, be able to achieve that within two weeks. Similarly, if a participant is attending a series of group education sessions to support weight management then the timescale has to relate to that specific outcome. This is important when reporting to those who have commissioned the service. They need to see that an education program is delivering outcomes in an appropriate and clearly specified time frame.

It is also appropriate to consider evaluating and revising the education session based on the evaluation and this will be covered in detail in Chapter 7.

4.8 How to deliver a training session

This will depend on the participants' needs, subject area, resources available, venue and facilitators. For more information on teaching methods and resources see Chapters 5 and 6. However, the choice of which teaching methods to use will be related to the target participants and the venue you are using. Here are some factors to consider.

Group size

As well as thinking about who will attend, it is important to think about the group size. The number of participants attending the session will influence the type of activity that you can include. Generally speaking, smaller classes allow for greater levels of interaction. The 'optimum' number of participants in a class is debatable and may in practice be determined by factors such as venue size, financial resources and number of available facilitators.

Teaching methods for target participants

Teaching methods should be appropriate for the characteristics of the group such as age, gender and culture. They should also consider more widely how confident and capable participants will be in contributing to discussion and activities. Taking into account the stages of group development as discussed in Chapter 8 can be helpful. For example, a newly formed group is unlikely to want to contribute to a philosophical debate about the causes of obesity but they might be happy to discuss what they know about high sugar foods.

Adult or child participants

How we learn as adults compared to when we were younger is also important to consider when planning education sessions. Whereas children are familiar with being sat in a classroom and engaging in learning activities, adults generally speaking are not. Adults have additional responsibilities and time pressures that often mean they may be impatient participants. Unlike children, adults also tend to be goal orientated and need to understand the relevance and benefits for themselves. They will be able to reflect, draw on their life experiences and use this to improve their understanding of the subject area, something that particularly younger children may not be able to do. Finally, adults are much more capable of being self-directed in their learning and should not need the same level of instruction from the facilitator.

Learning and teaching theory

This book is primarily about the facilitation of group education. However, it would not be appropriate to discuss delivering education sessions without making some reference to the relevant learning and teaching theory.

Firstly, it is important to think what we mean by the term 'learning'. Holli *et al.* (2014) describe learning as a change in a person as a result of an experience, an interaction with his or her environment or an interaction with another person. The change could be in knowledge, skills, attitudes, values and behaviours and would be relatively permanent outcomes. In group education for lifestyle change, we are looking for such changes (learning) to enable participants to apply the knowledge in a practical way (behaviour change). The challenge as facilitators is to work out how to give people the *right* experiences to support them to develop knowledge and skills to change behaviour. Facilitators need to be aware of their own preferences, strengths and weaknesses as it is likely that they will naturally choose to facilitate in a way that suits their own preferences. This may or may not be what is best for the participants. We do not all learn in the same way. There are many models and theories that are designed to help with understanding this and next are some examples that can be useful. In most cases facilitators will not have an opportunity to test the learning styles of individual participants. However, having an awareness of different learning preferences that participants might have allows the facilitator to include a variety of teaching methods that will hopefully engage participants.

VARK-Visual, Aural, Read/wRite, Kinaesthetic

The VARK questionnaire is based on the VARK guide to learning styles. Completing the questionnaire helps individuals to understand their learning preferences and suggests strategies that will enhance their learning. It was developed by Fleming in 1987 and has been used widely (Fleming and Mills, 1992). Some people have a very strong preference for one style or another whilst some may work well with a more mixed approach and are referred to as multimodal. A brief summary of the different learning preferences is given next:

- Visual (V). This refers to a preference to see information in a diagrammatic form such as spider diagrams, maps, graphs and flowcharts rather than in words. Parts of the diagram will be linked with arrows, circles or indication of the hierarchy. In group education using a whiteboard or flip chart to draw a diagram may help this type of learner. Diagrammatic representations of food groups such as the Eatwell Guide may be useful.
- Aural/auditory (A). This is a preference for information that is heard or spoken. In group education this will include listening to the facilitator, taking part in group discussion and speaking. Aural learners may repeat what has been said in their own words to reinforce their learning.
- Read/write (R). This is a preference for information presented as words and text based. In group education this includes written information such as that on presentations, handouts and leaflets. However, participants may also benefit when they are given an opportunity to write such as lists, goals for behaviour change, action plans and diaries (e.g. food intake or physical activity diaries).
- Kinaesthetic (K). This is the preference to use experience and practice to support learning. Participants will want to do something that relates the learning to reality. In group education this might include watching demonstrations or simulations of a 'real' situation, taking part in role plays, watching videos of real examples or completing case studies or other worked examples. Staff participants might practice explaining something to patients, service users or carers in a role play or work through a case study. Patient, service user or carer participants might practice obtaining information from food labels.

More detailed information and for access to the VARK questionnaire visit http://vark-learn.com.

Surface and deep learning

The idea of deep and surface learning comes from work completed by Marton and Saljo (1976a and b). People do not necessarily constantly learn in either a deep or a surface way although they may have a preference for one or the other. Their approach may relate to how motivated they are to learn the material. Surface learners might aim to learn facts and memorize information but may miss the point of how the learning can be applied to real life. Deep learning is going to be much more useful in group education in order to promote behaviour change, which needs to be a long-term approach if it is going to be effective. Deep learning will allow participants to understand and apply information into their daily life and experiences. Activities that encourage participants to think through the purpose of what they are learning and how it relates to their previous knowledge and experiences is more likely to support deep learning.

Honey and Mumford learning styles questionnaire
This is another commonly used learning style questionnaire with four learning styles identified. These are:
• Activists who are hands-on learners who like to have a go and learn by trial and error;
• Reflectors who like to be told what to do and have very clear explanations before they will attempt a task;
• Theorists who need to know why they need to do something and like to be reassured that it makes sense;
• Pragmatists who want to be shown what to do and see a demonstration from an expert.
More details about this can be found at www.peterhoney.com/. As with other theories of learning styles the key application for this in a group education session is to have a variety of teaching methods that are likely to meet the preferences of a range of learning styles and where possible use a four-point approach to the task. For example:
• a task needs to have a clear explanation (reflectors),
• to be demonstrated by an expert (pragmatist) such as the facilitator or perhaps an expert patient,
• to have a clear explanation as to why the task or recommended behaviour change is important (theorists) and
• an opportunity for participants to have a go (activists).
There are many other approaches to learning styles that are beyond the scope of this text but considering these increases the chance of all participants finding a task that supports their learning.

TOP TIP

Ensure that a variety of activities are included in the education session to increase the likelihood of the session supporting participant learning.

Writing a lesson plan

It is really important to have a clear plan of what is going to be done when and by whom when delivering group education sessions. In most cases there is a limited time frame to deliver the session. A clear lesson plan with timings helps with time management. It is also invaluable if more than one person is facilitating the session. Listing the resources needed for a particular part of the plan and noting which objectives are being delivered by which activity aids clarity. The following information is likely to be required for a comprehensive lesson plan:

- Description of the target audience
- Venue, date and time frame
- Aim and objectives of the session
- Participant learning outcomes
- An outline of the content of the session
- Descriptions of the learning activities that are to be undertaken (ideally these would be in sufficient detail for another experienced facilitator to deliver the session)
- Lists of resources required and facilities
- Timescales for individual components of the session
- Details of evaluation to be completed.

An example lesson plan is shown in Box 4.1, which indicates the type of material that it is useful to include. The detail of how these might be delivered and what could be included are covered in Chapter 5.

Box 4.1 Lesson plan

Name of Group: New Town Healthy Lifestyle Group   Number of participants: 10

Date: Tuesday 2nd February 2015   Time: 10 a.m.–12 noon

Venue: New Town Community Centre   Session number: 2 of 6

Session Leader: Sara-Jane Johnson, Community Dietitian

Session Title: Increasing physical activity.

Aim:

To empower participants to increase their physical activity level.

Objectives:

To inform participants of the current recommendations for physical activity
To identify reasons for physical inactivity
To empower participants to plan realistic ways to increase their physical activity level

Learning Outcomes:

By the end of the session, participants will:

1 Be able to state four benefits of regular physical activity
2 Have identified their current level of activity in relation to current recommendations
3 Have identified at least one personal barrier to undertaking regular physical activity
4 Be aware of at least three local services to access to increase activity
5 Have made an action plan of two things they will do over the next two weeks to increase their physical activity level

Resources:

Flip chart stand, paper and pens, refreshments, labels and pens for name badges, physical activity questionnaire, Health benefits of walking leaflet, Local Leisure Centre information, pedometers, Action Plan handout, Evaluation forms,

Time	Topic	Facilitator Activity	Participant Activity	Learning outcome
9.45–10.00		Preparation of room	None	
10–10.10	Welcome	Give name badges	Name badge refreshments	
10.10–10.20	Introduction	Recap on last week Aims and learning outcomes of this session	Listening	
10.20–10.30	Benefits of Physical activity	Facilitate group discussion on benefits of physical activity. Write responses on flip chart so all participants can see. Fill in gaps of what the group do not come up with.	Discussion	1
10.30–10.45	Recommendations for physical activity	Presentation of current physical activity recommendations Whole group discussion about these and what they mean in practical terms and how they can be achieved.	Discussion	2

(*Continued*)

10.45–11.00	Current levels of physical activity	Individual to complete physical activity questionnaire to identify current activity level in relation to current recommendations	Complete questionnaire	2
11.00–11.40	Increasing physical activity	Facilitate group discussion • What do people do now? • How do they feel about 'activity'? • What are the barriers? • How can we be more active? • Local Leisure Centre information, Health benefits of walking leaflet • Give out pedometers and explain	Group discussion Learning how to use pedometers	3 and 4
11.40–11.55	Action planning	Break out group discussion of possible actions and give out action plans for individuals to complete	Discussion Complete action plan	5
11.55–12	Summary and Evaluation	Summarize key points of the session Participant questions Give out evaluation forms	Completion of evaluation form	

References

Anderson LW, Krathwohl DR, Airasian PW, Cruikshank KA, Mayer RE *et al.* (2014). *A Taxonomy for Learning, Teaching and Assessing: A Revision of Bloom's. Pearson New International Edition*. Harlow: Pearson Education Limited.

Bloom BS (1956). *Taxonomy of Educational Objectives, Handbook I: The Cognitive Domain*. New York: David McKay Co Inc.

British Association for Cardiovascular Prevention and Rehabilitation (BACPR) (2012). *Standards and Core Components for Cardiovascular Disease Prevention and Rehabilitation*, 2nd Edn. [Online] Available from www.bacpr.com/resources/46c_bacpr_standards_and_core_components_2012.pdf [Accessed May 2016].

Cambridge Dictionaries [Online]. Available from: http://dictionary.cambridge.org/ [Accessed May 2016].

Department of Health (2010). *Maximising the Appeal of Weight Management Services*. London: HMSO.

East Midlands Health Trainer Hub (2014). *An Implementation Guide and Toolkit for Making Every Contact Count: Using Every Opportunity to Achieve Health and Wellbeing*.

Fleming ND and Mills C (1992). Not another inventory, rather a catalyst for reflection. *To Improve the Academy*, 11: 137–155. Available from: http://digitalcommons.unl.edu/podimproveacad/246 [Accessed May 2016].

Gillespie J, Midmore C, Hoeflich J, Ness C, Ballard P and Stewart L (2015). Parents as the start of the solution: a social marketing approach to understanding triggers and barriers to entering a childhood weight management service. *J Hum Nutr Diet* 28: 83–92.

Holli BB and Beto JA (2014). *Nutrition Counseling and Education Skills for Dietetics Professionals*, 6th Edn. Baltimore: Lippincott, Williams and Wilkins.

James DCS, Harville C, Efunbumi O and Martin MY (2015). Health literacy issues surrounding weight management among African American women: a mixed methods study. *J Hum Nutr Diet* 28(2): 41–49. Available from: DOI: 10.1111/jhn.12239. [Accessed November 2015].

Marton F and Saljo R (1976a). On qualitative differences in learning 1: Outcome and process. *Brit J Educ Psych* 46: 4–11.

Marton F and Saljo R (1976b). On qualitative differences in learning 2: Outcome as a function of the learner's conception of the task. *Brit J Educ Psych* 46: 115–127.

Naidoo J and Wills J (2009). *Foundations for Health Promotion*, 3rd Edn. London: Bailliere Tindall.

National Institute for Health and Care Excellence (2013). *Cardiac Rehabilitation Services NICE Commissioning Guide* [CMG40]. Available from: www.nice.org.uk/guidance/cmg40 [Accessed May 2016].

National Institute for Health and Care Excellence (NICE) (2014). Managing overweight and obesity in adults-lifestyle weight management services. Available from: www.nice.org.uk/guidance/ph53 [Accessed May 2016].

National Institute for Health and Care Excellence (NICE Pathways) (2015). Diabetes overview. Available from: http://pathways.nice.org.uk/pathways/diabetes [Accessed May 2016].

Further reading

http://vark-learn.com/
www.peterhoney.com/

Chapter 5 **Delivering the session**

Vanessa Halliday

5.1 Introduction

The focus of this chapter is on how group education sessions are delivered in practice. The chapter highlights the importance of making a positive start to the session and gives details and checklists for the type of information and activities that can be included. The discussion that follows covers a range of different educational activities and techniques that can be used to promote participant engagement and learning. The aim throughout is to give you practical examples and tips that will help you to facilitate interesting and effective education sessions that will promote lifestyle change.

5.2 Starting the session

Making sure that the start of the session goes well is important if you want to create a good first impression. Participants' motivation for attending will vary and whilst some will attend full of enthusiasm for what they are about to experience, others may be feeling apprehensive or even reluctant when they first walk through the door. If you are able to greet participants with a smile and engage in general welcoming conversation, this can help set the tone for the forthcoming session.

Arriving at the venue and preparation time

Arriving at the venue with time to prepare before participants enter is important and facilitators should plan for this. If you are driving to the venue unloading and transporting equipment, or even finding somewhere to park can take extra time that you hadn't anticipated. What needs to be done once inside will vary depending on the session but it could include getting rooms unlocked,

How to Facilitate Lifestyle Change: Applying Group Education in Healthcare, First Edition.
Amanda Avery, Kirsten Whitehead and Vanessa Halliday.
© 2017 John Wiley & Sons, Ltd. Published 2017 by John Wiley & Sons, Ltd.

putting up signs to direct people, rearranging furniture in the room, creating displays, setting up a computer and projector for presentations, sorting out refreshments and preparing for activities. Being disorganized when participants arrive can be stressful and appear unprofessional. It can also lead to a session starting late, which may lead to the need to reorganize content.

TOP TIPS FOR SEATING ARRANGEMENTS

Think about how you want the seating to be organized. If the chairs are in rows this may give the impression of a 'lecture' and that the participants are going to be given knowledge by the facilitator. It can also hinder group interaction and discussion. Other options include placing the seats in a 'U' shape facing the whiteboard or screen and facilitator. This arrangement means that participants can see each other more easily, leading to more interaction. If your aim is to remove hierarchy, you can place the chairs in a circle. The facilitator may then be seen as a member of the group. Depending on the activities that will be included it may be appropriate to seat the participants around tables. If this is the case, try to make sure that participants are able to face the facilitator when required as having to twist your body position can be uncomfortable.

Registration

In some cases, participants will need to sign in and be given resources or perhaps name badges, directed to toilet facilities or refreshments. This will not be relevant in every situation but should be considered.

Welcome and introductions

Introducing yourself to the group along with any co-facilitators that will be involved in the session is essential. It will also be helpful to explain a little about your background and how the education session came about. At this point you can introduce the session by giving an outline of the programme such as information on start and finish times and breaks. Some facilitators also choose to give an overview of the content, including the overall aim and objectives or learning outcomes and to hand out any resources. Others prefer to wait until after any icebreaker activities. Participants should be given the opportunity to ask any initial questions.

Unless the participants know each other well already, such as in a school class or a work department, it is good to have some opportunity for people to introduce themselves to each other too. Depending on your lesson plan you may choose to incorporate this into an icebreaker activity. Using name badges or desk name cards can prevent facilitators and participants from having to memorize everyone's name.

Housekeeping

There are always some housekeeping arrangements to make participants aware of and these should be clarified at the beginning of the session. These could include the following:

- Venue layout and location of toilets
- Fire escapes and meeting point; whether a fire alarm is expected or not
- If and where smoking areas are located
- Room comfort such as heating or air conditioning temperature
- Refreshment breaks and catering facilities
- Security issues such as locking rooms, which is particularly relevant if participants are likely to move to breakout rooms
- Safe keeping of valuables
- Respect for copyright of materials.

Icebreakers

In some sessions, particularly when participants are unfamiliar with each other, it may help to undertake an icebreaker activity. Icebreakers can help participants to get to know one another, help integrate new members, encourage participants to cooperate and work together, help people feel more at ease and create a good atmosphere for learning and participation. When deciding which icebreaker to use there are a number of factors to consider as the activity needs to be appropriate and something that everyone can get involved in. Consider participant characteristics such as age, gender, familiarity within the group, intellectual ability, cultural differences, mobility and likely knowledge base. Practically, you should also take into account the size of the group, space, resources and time. The amount of time taken on an icebreaker should relate to the length of the education session. If you only have an hour, then the icebreaker should only take a few minutes. Don't allow icebreakers to go on for too long as participants can lose interest. You can be as creative as you like with icebreakers but you may wish to choose something that is linked to the programme in some way rather than purely as a way of getting to know each other.

To encourage participant engagement in the icebreaker be enthusiastic and introduce the activity by telling the group why you are doing it. Follow this up with clear instructions of what participants need to do and how long they have. Ideally, instructions should be given verbally and written on a slide, whiteboard or flip chart. If you can give an example, this can help. Facilitate the activity by controlling the time. This is particularly important if participants need to swap over during the discussion or rotate around the group. Think about if and how you want participants to feedback to the

Table 5.1 Examples of 'getting to know you' icebreakers.

Icebreaker	Instructions
People bingo	Prepare the bingo cards in advance by drawing a grid (e.g. four by four) on a piece of paper. In each box in the grid write a statement such as 'plays a musical instrument', 'has a pet dog', 'plays tennis', 'name begins with A', 'can speak Spanish'. Distribute a card to each participant and ask them to circulate around the group, introducing themselves to others and asking the questions on the card. Once they have found someone who matches the description they should ask them to sign the box. You can continue the activity for, for example 10 minutes or until someone has a row of four signatures, in which case they should shout 'BINGO'.
Interviews	Ask the participants to work in pairs. They should then be given two to three minutes each to introduce themselves and 'interview' the other person to find out three interesting facts that they can then feedback to the whole group.
Desert island	Ask participants to consider the following 'If you were to be cast away on a desert island (1) what one luxury item, (2) what book and (3) what piece of music would you want with you? Participants should be given two to three minutes to write down their list before sharing it with the whole group.
Time machine	Ask participants to consider the following 'If you had a time machine what year would you go to and why?' Participants should be given two to three minutes to write down their response before sharing it with the whole group.
True or false	Ask participants to write down three facts about themselves that they are happy to disclose to the group. Two of the facts should be true and one false. Participants should then take it in turns to read out their list and other group members should decide and vote on which are true and false.
Art work	Particularly if you are working with groups of children you could use an icebreaker that involves drawing a picture. For example, this could be a self-portrait, their family or their favourite game.

whole group. At the very least, there should be the opportunity for a brief debrief and for participants to make any comments or ask questions. Table 5.1 gives examples of icebreaker activities and how to organize them.

Exploring hopes, fears and expectations
Participants coming to education sessions come with a variety of thoughts and beliefs about what is going to happen; some of these will be positive and some negative. Some participants may have been pressurized into attending

Table 5.2 Examples of hopes, fears and expectations.

Hopes	Fears	Expectations (positive and negative)
To gain new information	I won't have anything to say	I'm going to learn something useful
To meet people 'like me'	I might talk too much	I'm not going to learn anything from this session
To find someone who understands my condition	I might say something stupid or make a fool of myself	It will be boring
To have fun	Everyone else knows more than me	It will be interesting
To learn new skills	What if no-one will talk to me?	The facilitator will be professional
To find ways to cope better with my illness	There might be role-play	We will finish on time
To find some motivation to change my lifestyle	I'm really tired, I hope I don't fall asleep	It's a waste of time me being here

and be resistant to engaging, some may have very high expectations of what the session is going to enable them to do. On some occasions the expectations may be unrealistic or participants may be misinformed about what the session is going to deliver. All of this needs to be managed by the facilitator and spending some time exploring participant views can help clarify the reality of what is planned but also allow the facilitator, if they are able, to try and adjust the content to address participant questions. Table 5.2 shows examples of some common hopes, fears and expectations that participants may have. Asking participants to talk in pairs or small groups and then feeding back to the whole group can increase participants' confidence in airing their views. Finding that other people have similar fears or anxieties can be supportive.

This might also be an appropriate time in your lesson plan for you to ask participants if they have any expectations about what is going to be covered in the session, or any questions that they are hoping to have answered. Making a note of these on the flip chart, referring back to them as the session progresses, as well as ensuring that they have been addressed at the end, is a good way of ensuring the content has been participant focussed.

Ground rules or agreement for working together

It is easy to assume that people know what to expect and how to behave in an education session but this may not be the case and spending a few minutes identifying what is important to that group, and the facilitator, can mean that all participants 'sign up' to the agreement. This will hopefully mean that there will be fewer difficulties later in the session. Making a record of what is discussed and posting it up in the room can act as an ongoing reminder. The agreement should be group led and asking participants to think of positive and negative past experiences can help generate ideas. Examples to consider include:

- Time keeping (facilitator(s) and participants)
- How are people expected to behave?
- Participants are expected to engage and contribute
- All should treat each other with respect
- Listening to other participant viewpoints and not interrupting
- No-one should dominate the group discussions
- Observing confidentiality, that is, what is shared in the session should not be shared outside of the group
- What is the expectation with mobile phones?
- What should people do if they are late?

5.3 Educational activities

Irrespective of whether you are working with groups of adults or children, using methods that encourage participants to actively engage in the session are most likely to be effective in promoting lifestyle change. For this reason, the educational activities discussed in this chapter will promote active learning. The traditional 'lecture' (where the participants are passive in the experience in that they enter the room, listen and absorb the information, then leave) will not be included. Educationalists agree that this type of session is likely to lead to participants adopting a surface, or superficial, approach to their learning (Exley, 2010) that, within the context of this book, is unlikely to encourage sustained lifestyle change.

TOP TIP FOR CAPTURING KEY LEARNING POINTS

Educational activities that promote active learning and participant engagement can, and hopefully do, lead to participants experiencing an 'Ah-ha!' moment. This may be a sudden understanding of what was thought to be an incomprehensible problem or where 'the penny drops' and they suddenly understand 'why'. Providing participants with a card at the start of the session (ideally coloured so it doesn't get lost with all the other course materials) to write down as the session progresses their 'Ah-ha!' moments, along with any other key learning points, can be a good way to ensure these are not forgotten.

Presentation slides

Most of you will be familiar, either as a facilitator or a participant, with education sessions that have been delivered using presentation slides. These are most commonly developed using tools such as PowerPoint, Prezi or Keynote. Using slides can be an incredibly useful way of structuring the session and communicating key messages to the participants. However, used in isolation slides can result in a passive education style with minimal participant interaction. To avoid slipping into delivering a 'lecture', include individual and group activities throughout the presentation.

TOP TIPS FOR USING PRESENTATION SLIDES

- Keep the amount of text on each slide to a minimum. As a guide, include up to five or six points only. The text should reinforce what you are saying rather than repeat it word for word.
- Vary the format by including a variety of text and other graphics such as diagrams, pictures or tables. Avoid placing text over an image as it makes it difficult to read.
- Choose the background and font colour carefully. A light background and dark font or vice versa works well. Some colours and combinations such as red, green and yellow are not easy to read.
- The font style should be simple and easy to read, for example, sans serif such as Arial or Verdana. A font point size of 28+ should mean that it can be read from a distance.
- Avoid over-ambitious graphics such as words or images zooming in from all directions as this can be distracting.
- If you are using audio, graphics or hyperlinks make sure these work before the session begins. Use of hyperlinks will require the equipment you are using to be connected to the internet. Remember that using a wireless connection may result in slower download speed which may be an issue, particularly if you are using video or audio.
- Make sure you are familiar with the presentation software that you are using. Practice beforehand as required.

Use of questions

As a facilitator, integrating questions into your education session can be useful for a number of reasons. First and foremost, asking the group a question can help you to ascertain the level of baseline knowledge on the subject area and can be a good indicator of the group's understanding of what has been covered. Questions can also encourage participation and engagement. Used

Table 5.3 Types of questions that can be incorporated into an education session.

Question type	Purpose	Examples
Direct closed questions with right or wrong answers	Answers demonstrate level of knowledge and understanding of the participant that responds	Often factual and include how, what, where, when and who. 'How many calories are there in one gram of fat?'
Participant polls	Gives an opportunity for all participants to engage and respond	'Raise your hand if you agree with...' 'Raise your hand if you disagree with...'
Discussion generating open questions	Allows participants to share experiences and to learn from and support each other	'What is your experience of...?' 'What is your opinion on...?' 'What are your thoughts on...?'
Evaluative	Although there may be a factual element to the response, participants are able to expand on their answer	'What are the differences between...?' 'What are the similarities between...?' 'Can you describe...?'
Probing questions	Encourages participants to think and reflect in more depth	'What exactly do you mean by that?' 'Can you explain in more detail about...?' 'What is it that brings you to that conclusion?'

appropriately they can stimulate discussion and give valuable insight into participants' experiences and opinions. It may be that some of the questions that you ask are included in your lesson plan and have a direct link to a learning outcome, other may be more spontaneous. Whether planned or not, how you ask the questions needs some consideration. Examples of the different types of questions that can be asked are shown in Table 5.3.

When asking questions, it is important that they are clear and concise. Vague questions have the potential to remain unanswered or may mean that the discussion goes off at a tangent. Loaded and leading questions should also be avoided unless you only want participants to say what you want to hear. Equally, try to ask only one question at a time as this will prevent confusion as to what participants are meant to be thinking about and responding to. Particularly when asking discussion generating and probing questions such as those included in Table 5.3, make sure that you allow enough time for the group to think about what they want to say. It is too often the case that facilitators, not wanting there to be silence in the room, jump in and answer their own question. If there is no response after a minute or so, try rephrasing the question.

Encouraging participation is an essential part of facilitating group education. This means that participants need to feel comfortable and confident when contributing. One way to encourage this is to refrain from saying that a response to a question is wrong. Instead, if their answer is inaccurate or unclear, use probing questions such as 'that's interesting, what is it that brings you to that conclusion?' or 'can you give us an example?'

TOP TIP FOR INCLUSIVE FACILITATION

Try to invite all members of the group to respond to questions. One technique for this is to make eye contact with different people when asking different questions. Alternatively, you can specifically ask for answers from a certain part of the room, for example, towards the back of the room. This can help avoid the same person dominating throughout the session.

Discussion

Like questions, a discussion will encourage participant engagement and should help facilitate group directed education and learning. On an individual level, this type of activity will give members the opportunity to explore things in more depth, allowing opinions and experiences to be voiced. It can also help people to work through some of their own beliefs and potential misconceptions. On a group level, discussion can enable an individual to consider an alternative viewpoint or reassure others that may be thinking the same thing or who have had similar experiences. Importantly, discussion can encourage group members to support each other to understand and learn more about themselves and their situation.

Asking a question may well turn into a discussion and this may or may not have been your intention. Spontaneous discussion may be extremely useful but, if not factored into the lesson plan, it may be at the expense of an alternative activity or content. Alternatively, techniques such as brainstorming can be an effective way of generating discussion across the whole group.

Brainstorming

A brainstorming activity can be incorporated into any education session irrespective of group size. Indeed, it can be a useful tool when you want to encourage participant engagement and interaction in larger groups.

The activity should begin with a question or problem being posed by the facilitator. One option is then to ask the group for their answers and ideas. Alternatively, in order to give participants time to think, a few minutes can be allocated for them to make notes of their thoughts individually or to discuss them with the person sat next to them. You can then write down either on a whiteboard or flip chart answers that are generated by the group. One idea to encourage active participation by all group members is to go around each member of the group asking for one answer or idea. To avoid the anxiety that this might cause some quieter members of the group, this is better done after participants have had the chance to discuss their ideas with others. If you have already thought about what ideas might be raised, you can begin to structure what you are writing into themes. Alternatively, you might want to write them down randomly and ask the group to summarize the meaning. Rather than writing them down yourself you can ask for one of the participants to volunteer as the scribe. When the answers dry up use prompts such as 'Have you thought about…?' or 'What about…?' to generate more until you believe you have reached saturation. Importantly, at the end of the activity you need to summarize the points that have been discussed. This may also include highlighting where incorrect or inappropriate answers have been made. Care needs to be taken not to alienate the participant that raised that particular point so this needs to be managed in a supportive way. This tends to be made easier when there are a number of responses that are inaccurate or misconstrued as they can then be discussed collectively. Indeed, it may be that you prefer to gently challenge inappropriate responses when they are said rather than noting them down on the board. This can also avoid participants making notes that could be misinterpreted at a later date.

Brainstorming is a great activity for generating and sharing ideas in a short amount of time. However, if your aim is to generate a deeper level of discussion to more complex questions and scenarios, using breakout group discussion based activities might be more fruitful.

How to facilitate discussion based breakout group activities

1 For a planned discussion based breakout group activity make sure that there is a well-defined objective to the task.
2 Give clear instructions verbally and written as to what the discussion question(s) is.
3 As for any breakout group activity, decide if you want the participants to allocate themselves to a group or if there are reasons why facilitator-allocated groups would work better. This may be the case if the discussion would be enhanced by having group members with certain characteristics

or experience, where certain members of the group have well-established relationships or where you have already identified the potential for conflict within the group.

4 Decide if you want all groups to discuss the same question or different ones.

5 Allocate a realistic amount of time for the activity. Unless it is a short and simple question, 5 minutes is not likely to be long enough whereas 30 minutes may result in disengagement and boredom from some group members. Inform the groups how long they have and announce when, for example half the time has elapsed, or when there are only 5 minutes remaining.

6 Identify how the key points from each breakout group will be fed back to the whole group. Do you want them to write down a summary on flip chart paper? Do they need to appoint a group 'spokesperson'? Time permitting, allow as many members of the group the opportunity to participate in the feedback.

7 Whilst the activity is in progress keep the groups focussed and make sure that the discussion doesn't go off at a tangent. Walk around the room and spend a few minutes listening to each of the group's discussion. Where necessary encourage participation from the quieter members of the group. Watch for signs that the discussion is deteriorating into either a heated debate or chat about social weekend activities. Where this is happening, facilitate getting the group back on track or, if it is across all groups, either all that needs to be said has been said or possibly the instructions weren't clear enough.

8 During the debrief or feedback, take notes and at the end summarize the key points that have been raised and what the conclusion was, if indeed there was one. Ideally this can be done on a whiteboard or flip chart. Identify any areas that have been missed but avoid taking over the feedback yourself. During the session use positive verbal (yes, great, good idea) and non-verbal (nods, smiles) encouragement.

Buzz groups

You may be familiar with the term 'buzz groups'. In essence, a buzz group is a discussion based breakout group activity that usually involves participants working in pairs or small groups, discussing a question for a few minutes, then feeding back to the whole group. Like other discussion based activities, buzz groups engage participants, are good for stimulating and generating ideas, sharing experiences or opinions, as well as allowing time for thinking and reflection for both participants and facilitators.

TOP TIP FOR DETERMINING BREAKOUT GROUP SIZE

Think about what the ideal group size is to best achieve the desired learning outcome. For example, asking individuals to complete a task may allow time for personal reflection but could result in anxiety around having to 'present back' individual thoughts to the wider group. Asking participants to work in pairs or trios can be effective in allowing more detailed discussion and gives quieter participants an opportunity to contribute. Whilst groups of between 4 and 10 people still allow for sharing of ideas and experiences, beyond this there is increased likelihood of disengagement of timid or more reticent members and more chance of the group fragmenting.

Using multimedia (audio, text and video clips)

In addition to simply posing a question for discussion, alternative discussion-based activities can be developed around a range of multimedia resources such as audio, video, photographs, magazine or newspaper articles. Whilst a photograph can capture a moment in time, audio and in particular video clips, can be a more powerful way of illustrating a key message in your education session as they often give a real-world relevance to what is being discussed. Alternatively, you could choose to use video or a pre-recorded session to demonstrate a task such as cooking or exercise. There are numerous video resources available online. Selecting the appropriate one is important so watch it through several times beforehand to be confident that it is delivering the correct message. Although many are free to use with the appropriate Creative Commons license (see Chapter 6 for further details), this is something that you need to check out. You should also be aware of commercially produced media resources that might contain advertisements.

As with other activities, if you are going to use multimedia resources, give an explanation about its purpose before you start. For example, if you are using audio or video, include a brief overview of what the clip is about, how long it will play for and what will happen at the end in terms of discussion. Most of all, be clear about what you want the participants to get out of it. Do you want them to read, watch or listen for something in particular or are there questions that you would like them to answer at the end? You can decide if the ensuing discussion will happen as the whole group, or if it would be better to first get the participants to reflect in smaller breakout groups. If you are asking them to read a long article, or if the video runs for more than 5–6 minutes, you might want to consider breaking it into sections with discussion at the intervals. This can prevent some members of the group getting distracted or losing focus.

Importantly, if you are using audio or video, before you start the session check to make sure that the sound and picture quality are good and you know how to work the equipment. Rather than relying on internet download speeds, if you can, pre-load it onto the hard drive of the computer or a USB flash drive. If you are in an unfamiliar venue and have not had chance before the day of the session to check out the equipment, you might want to consider having an alternative plan, just in case of the exceptional occurrence when it will not play.

TOP TIP FOR QUESTIONS AND DISCUSSIONS

Make sure that everyone in the group can hear what has been said by other participants. If in doubt check, then either ask for them to repeat it or paraphrase their response yourself.

Role play and simulation

Role play and simulation activities involve the play-acting of an imaginary scenario. It is something that most of us will have experience of at one time or another. Whether this was as a child playing make believe or as an adult running through the 'what if?' scenarios of how an event may develop and turn out. Whereas during simulation activities the participants are acting and responding as themselves, in role play they take on the role of a made-up character. There are a number of ways that role play and simulation can be incorporated into education sessions.

Role play using facilitators or actors

Using facilitators or actors to role play a scenario can have a powerful effect on an individual's understanding of a situation and the impact of lifestyle change. For example, two opposing scenarios of how an individual makes changes (or not) to their behaviour can be acted out. During the first, the individual is in a consultation with their doctor receiving the good news that their latest medical investigations have shown that their BMI, cholesterol and heart attack risk have all reduced. The opposing scenario is that the individual is in hospital following a near fatal heart attack. These scenarios could be extended to include family members so that the impact of ill health is demonstrated at a wider level.

The group observing the role play should be advised to identify not only what the underlying impact of the conversation is but also what emotions are being expressed and what the long term implications of such a scenario could be. Whilst you may have access to amateur or professional actors that will ensure that the scenario is performed consistently and to a high standard, the cost of this may be prohibitive. For this reason, you may choose to ask other facilitators or colleagues to be involved in the role play activity.

Group participant role play and simulation

Rather than using actors or facilitators, role play and simulation can involve members of the group working together to act out a scenario. The number of people involved in the scenario may vary but, for example, could include two people conversing whilst the third person keeps time, observes and take notes. Roles within the group can then be rotated.

Role play activities could include scenarios with, for example, health professionals or teachers, such as the one described previously. Alternatively, as outlined in Table 5.4, you could ask participants to use either simulation or role play to act out the scene.

If you are involved in educating staff you may wish to develop scenarios that give them the opportunity to practice their communication skills and dialogue. Examples include discussing smoking cessation advice with a client or how to broach difficult conversations with more reluctant individuals, such as reducing alcohol intake or weight management. Video recording the role play activity and then watching it back with the individuals can be a powerful way to enhance their learning. However, this type of activity needs

Table 5.4 Examples of role play and simulation scenarios.

Lifestyle behaviour	Scenario
Increasing physical activity	1. Discussion between friends, or with a partner, how you will increase your physical activity level. 2. Discussion between friends, or with a partner, how you will overcome perceived barriers (e.g. time, equipment) to engaging in more physical activity.
Weight management	1. How to say no when offered an additional portion/cake/biscuit/sweets/snacks in the workplace or at a friend or relative's house. 2. How to refuse dessert when out for a meal.
Stopping smoking	1. Resisting social pressure of being offered a cigarette at a party/bar/friend's house. 2. Rehearsing the discussion with a healthcare worker about seeking support to give up smoking.
Moderating alcohol intake	1. How to say no when offered a drink at a party/bar/or at home.

careful facilitation as for some individuals watching themselves on TV can be quite challenging. To improve their confidence and skills, ensuring that the discussion starts with and focusses on what they did well, as well as highlighting areas for development, is vital.

No matter how enthusiastically you introduce a role play or simulation activity there may still be some members of the group who groan. It is possible that participants may have had a previous negative experience and are reluctant to engage. Exploring expectations and addressing these concerns prior to the activity can help overcome this. In addition to this, for some individuals, certain scenarios may be emotive, resulting in them becoming distressed or upset. This can be avoided by advising participants before the activity begins to use scenarios that are not familiar to them. There should also be an opportunity for an individual to opt out of the activity if they wish. In some cases, providing onward referrals to external support agencies may be required.

Fishbowl role play
An alternative method to using group participant role play is using the Fishbowl technique. This method gets its name from the arrangement of the group seating, with two or more chairs positioned opposite each other in the centre of the room with all other group members sitting in a circle around them. The role play takes place in the centre, observed by the rest of the group who then give feedback and discuss what happened.

TOP TIPS FOR EFFECTIVE ROLE PLAY AND SIMULATION ACTIVITIES

- Take time to explain the aim and objectives of the activity as this will help give focus to the group.
- Keep the scenarios simple and choose scenarios that are relevant and realistic to the group. Where possible get the group to identify what scenarios they want to role play or simulate.
- Give clear verbal and written instructions about what to do and what the scenario is.
- If you are using group participant role play, consider demonstrating one of the scenarios first. This is particularly important if group members are unlikely to have done it before.
- Reassure group members that are apprehensive and anxious. Give the group an opt out option if anyone feels completely unable to participate.

- For the Fishbowl technique, ask for volunteers from the group rather than selecting individuals who may be reluctant.
- Circulate around the room as the activity progresses to make sure participants understand the task and keep focussed. Or, if using the Fishbowl technique, you may wish to stop the role play and ask questions about what is happening and then continue.
- All role play and simulation activities should include a group discussion and debrief where any ideas, issues or concerns that have come up can be discussed with the whole group.
- End with a summary from either the group or the facilitators of the main learning points.
- Manage the time. This is particularly important where roles need to be rotated as with the group participant activities. You need to ensure that there is enough time for the group discussion and learning points.

Case studies

Case studies are stories or scenarios that can bridge the gap between theory and real life, helping participants to relate to the subject being discussed. They can be incorporated into an education session either by the facilitator talking through and referring to the case, or as a group activity. The latter will give participants the opportunity to understand and discuss the case in more depth. If you are writing your own case study include enough detail to make it interesting and engaging without being overly complex. Alternatively, providing you maintain complete anonymity, you may have real life cases that you can use.

Box 5.1 gives an example of the type of case study that you could include as a group activity. There are a number of ways that you could focus the discussion from this scenario. For example, what are Mr Harris' health risks; what lifestyle factors contribute to this risk; what are the potential barriers to Mr Harris changing his lifestyle and how could these be overcome? Alternatively, you may wish to include further information on dietary intake that can be critiqued or a menu planning activity for participants to complete.

Case studies are a useful tool in supporting participants to consider alternative viewpoints so if this is your aim make sure that there is more than one possible answer. There may be diverse opinions about how the scenario could be managed, or what the solutions might be, so be prepared to facilitate what could be a heated discussion.

> **Box 5.1** Case study example
>
> Bob Harris is a 53-year-old gentleman who works full time as a salesman. Mr Harris is married and has two teenage children, Samantha (13 years) and Peter (15 years). His wife works as a nurse in his local doctor's surgery. Mr Harris' job means that he often travels around the country and has to stay in hotels two to three nights most weeks. Recently, Mr Harris has been feeling more tired than usual and is getting out of breath when walking up stairs. When he visited his doctor 6 weeks ago, the following measurements were recorded: body mass index 38 kg/m^2 (obese); blood pressure 145/90 mmHg (hypertension); cholesterol 6.9 mmol/L (hypercholesterolae-mia); alcohol intake 25 units a week; does not smoke.
>
> Example discussion points for participants:
> - What are Mr Harris' health risks?
> - What lifestyle factors contribute to this risk?
> - What are the potential barriers to Mr Harris changing his lifestyle and how could these be overcome?
> - How could Mr Harris incorporate physical activity into his lifestyle?

Demonstrations and active participation

Many group education sessions aimed at facilitating lifestyle change are likely to include a demonstration such as cooking or physical activity. There are many advantages of using a 'live' demonstration such as being able to adapt what you are doing, and your explanations, to the needs of the participants. You can also stop, start and repeat steps and answer questions as the demonstration progresses. Depending on your lesson plan, you may choose to get the group actively participating in the activity. If this is the case, you will need to make sure that they have arrived at the session prepared. For example, if you are asking them to take part in physical activity, they will need to be wearing appropriate clothing and footwear. You will also need to give careful consideration to how many participants should be in the group. This may well be linked to a risk assessment and how many facilitators are available to supervise. In some cases, it might be appropriate to give participants the opportunity to 'opt out' of the activity.

The organization and running of, for example, a cookery demonstration is challenging, particularly if this is not something that you are experienced in. The following tips are related to a demonstration, such as a 'Cook and Eat' session, but may also be helpful when planning other similar activities.

TOP TIPS FOR A SUCCESSFUL COOKERY DEMONSTRATION

Before the session:

- Choose your recipe carefully. First and foremost, make sure that it is appropriate for the nutritional messages you want to convey. Other things to think about include the cost of ingredients for your budget and for participants, how available the ingredients are locally (are they in season), are they culturally acceptable and will participants have the cooking skills and equipment to prepare the dish at home. You will also need to make sure that the dish is not too complicated and that you will have time to cook it and clear away within the allotted time.
- Think about how you will structure the demonstration. If the participants are also going to be cooking the dish would it be better to demonstrate the initial preparation stages, get them to go and do it then come back and observe a demonstration of the next stage and so on. When will be the best time to discuss, for example, the healthy eating messages related to the session? This could be whilst the dish is cooking or at the end following tasting. Don't forget to factor in set-up and clear-up time.
- Prepare recipe cards for participants, making sure the instructions are in enough detail and ideally laminating them so that they can be wiped clean.
- Practice the demonstration a few times noting down the equipment that you are using. Make the dish following the recipe written on the card.
- Be familiar with the venue where you will be doing the demonstration, particularly in terms of what equipment will be there and what you need to take with you. Don't rely on what was there on your previous visit as it may have changed. Make sure you are familiar with how to use the appliances.
- Write a comprehensive equipment list. Don't forget that you may also need to provide utensils for tasting and containers for participants to take home what they have prepared. Think about food safety regulations too. Do you need to take hand-sanitizer, food temperature probes and a first aid kit?
- Your shopping list should take into account the number of portions of the dish that will be prepared along with any other ancillary items such as waste bags and cleaning products. If the participants are also cooking the dish, you may wish to include a little extra in case of any mishaps.
- Purchase the ingredients in advance of the session. If you leave it to the day you may run into difficulties if the store that you go to is out of stock. If you buy them too early there may be issues around 'use by' dates. How will you transport and store ingredients that need to be kept chilled?

- Do you need to do a risk assessment including first aid procedures and accident reporting? Have you and the other facilitators got the appropriate food hygiene qualifications?
- Having a list of resources for the session can be really helpful, particularly if the session is likely to be repeated.

On the day of the session:

- Arrive in advance of the session starting. One to two hours should allow plenty of time for unloading of the equipment and setting up of the demonstration.
- Decide if you are going to pre-weigh the ingredients or include this as you go along. Some participants may not have weighing scales at home and may need to be shown how to use them. They may also require handy measures to be used instead.
- If you are using the oven(s), what time do they need turning on?

During the demonstration:

- Introduce the demonstration by, for example, giving an explanation of the dish and why it has been chosen. Repeat the key nutritional messages at different stages of the demonstration.
- If you are using a recipe card, hand copies out to the participants. Follow the stages as they are written on the card to avoid confusion when participants are cooking the dish.
- Follow the appropriate food hygiene regulations. For example, hair should be tied back, fingernails should be short and nail polish removed and you should wear appropriate clothing, closed-in shoes and an apron. Pay close attention to your hand washing technique as well as appropriate use of, for example, chopping boards.
- Explain each of the ingredients that you will be using. This may be before you start or as you incorporate them into the recipe. You may also want to explain the equipment and how to use it.
- Keep a close eye on the time. This is particularly important if the dish requires a minimum cooking time.
- For tasting of the dish use small pots or dishes rather than risking dipping of spoons that have already been eaten from.
- Decide what you want to do with leftover food and ingredients and try and avoid waste.

After the session:

- Make sure you factor in enough time for cleaning up after the demonstration has finished. This will include washing up, cleaning down work surfaces and getting rid of waste. If you are using a dishwasher you will need to agree who will empty it and put away the equipment.

Games

Games can be used as an effective educational tool and can be a fun way to incorporate active learning into your session. Whereas some games will be designed to improve participants' knowledge, others can be used to develop cognitive and decision-making skills. Although commonly associated with educating children, games can be used for all age groups. Ensuring that they are age appropriate and could not be perceived as childish or patronizing by older participants is, however, important. Before you incorporate a game into your lesson plan make sure that you have played it from start to finish so that you are clear about the instructions, you know how long it takes and importantly, you are aware what you expect participants to learn from taking part. Some games such as electronic games or apps, that incorporate, for example role playing and simulation, will be played individually. Other more traditional board or card games can be played by everyone or smaller breakout groups. Giving clear instructions and a post-game debrief is also necessary. Examples of games will be given in Chapter 6.

Quizzes and questionnaires

There are a number of reasons why you may choose to include a quiz or questionnaire in your lesson plan. For example, a knowledge-based quiz can help the facilitator determine participants' existing understanding or, if presented later on in the session, it can be an indicator of what they have learnt. Other self-assessment questionnaires may be related to behaviour, personality or interests. Whilst some participants will find this type of activity fun, others may lack confidence and feel challenged. For this reason, if you are writing your own questions, you may wish to include some that are easy to answer and others that are more challenging. You should also consider the impact of telling participants that there will be quiz. If it is knowledge based, some people will feel that they are being tested and be anxious about this. Asking participants to complete this types of activity in pairs is one way to overcome this. However, behaviour focussed questionnaires are generally better completed by the individual and, depending on the types of questions being asked, it may help to make it clear that responses will not be shared across the group. The case studies in Chapter 6 include some examples of quizzes and questionnaires that are available for you to use.

Audience response systems

If you do choose to include a quiz or survey in your session an alternative to doing this as a paper-based activity is to use an audience response system. This will allow participants in the group to interact in the session and anonymously answer questions.

There are two main ways that you can do this. The first uses audience response computer software and hardware such as Meridia, Qwizdom and TurningPoint, that allows you to build multiple choice questions into your presentation slides. Each participant is given a wireless keypad that they use to click on what they believe to be the correct answer to the question. Answers are collected by a receiver attached to the computer, collated and shown on the projection screen. The alternative is to use cloud based audience response software or mobile polling apps that allow participants to respond to questions using their own mobile devices. This does of course mean that you have to be confident that everyone has a charged, wirelessly connected mobile device, or that you provide one for them to use during the session.

Self-directed out-of-session activities

Depending on the type of education session, it may be appropriate to ask participants to engage in a pre-session activity. This could be as simple as reading through an article or completing a questionnaire. Alternatively, it may be more time consuming such as keeping a food diary or filling in a self-reflection questionnaire relating to health behaviours. If there is more than one session in the series, between session activities may also be appropriate. Importantly, along with the instructions, you need to make it clear what the purpose of the activity is. You should also include time in the session for a debrief as, without this, participants may feel that they have wasted their time. Don't be surprised if some members of the group have not completed the task and, where appropriate, encourage them to engage with the activity at a later date.

Using the internet for group education

Over the last decade the number of people that use the internet has tripled with around 40% of the world's population now getting online each day (Internet Statistics Live, 2015). The percentage of the population that has internet access varies across the globe. For example, in high income countries such as the UK and USA, around 85 to 90% of the population have internet access. This is in contrast with some of the low and middle income areas of the world where between 20% and 50% of the population are connected (Internet Statistics Live, 2015). Depending on where in the world you are working, it is likely that a significant proportion of the participants attending your group education sessions will have internet access.

Alongside a change in the number of internet users, the way that we use the world wide web has also diversified. Whilst many of us will access websites to read, watch videos and learn about subjects that take our interest there are increasingly many other features of the internet, such as blogs, social networking sites, media sharing and live 'chat' functions that enable us to interact with the content and with each other online. As the internet has grown in popularity, unsurprisingly, its use within health has begun to be explored. Indeed 'e-health' as a term, has been around since the late 1990s.

Definition of e-health (Eysenbach, 2001):

> 'e-health is an emerging field in the intersection of medical informatics, public health and business, referring to health services and information delivered or enhanced through the internet and related technologies. In a broader sense, the term characterizes not only a technical development, but also a state-of-mind, a way of thinking, an attitude, and a commitment for networked, global thinking, to improve healthcare locally, regionally, and worldwide by using information and communication technology.'

Along with efficiency, enhancing quality, evidence based, empowerment, encouragement, enabling, extending, ethics and equity, education is, as described by Eysenbach (2001), one of the 10 'e's in e-health. However, in practice, the evidence base that supports the use of the internet in health education is still somewhat in its infancy and largely focusses on individual participant interventions and use of the internet to facilitate peer to peer support (Lal and Adair, 2014; Pal et al., 2014) rather than group education per se.

Examples of how the internet and social media can be used to support group education sessions

There are a number of ways that the internet can be used to support group education. As discussed earlier in this chapter, you may choose to include multimedia internet resources such as links to websites, audio and video clips during the education session. Other ways that the internet can be used include:

- Advertising and informing potential participants about the education session
- Posting pre and mid-session activities such as goal setting tasks online
- Using the internet as a repository for online resources
- Posting evaluation surveys online
- Providing ongoing support for participants that have attended by creating virtual communities for peer to peer, or ongoing motivational support from the facilitator.

Web pages and websites

The easiest way to get the information related to your education session online is to add content or a web page to an existing organizational website. The website could be owned, for example, by your employer or a local branch of a charity or patient support group. The first step will be for you to find out who the Webmaster is and, if they are happy to post your information, you will need to send them a document that includes exactly what details you want adding. Where there is no organizational website that you can use you may choose to set up your own. If you are new to website design and development, using a content management system such as WordPress, Google sites or Drupal will make the website much more manageable to build and maintain. Having support from an IT specialist or learning technologist will ensure that the website is fit for purpose.

In addition to providing practical information about the education session such as time, location and how to sign up to attend you can also provide links to additional multimedia resources and other websites. You may also wish to add a discussion forum where people can post questions or comments.

Social networking

Social networking sites such as Facebook, MySpace or Google + can be used to create a virtual community where participants can connect, ask questions and share their experiences. Facilitators can also share information and add supportive and motivational posts for members of the group.

Blogs

A blog can be an interesting and effective way of keeping people informed with information and events. If you are thinking about setting up a blog decide what the purpose is and who it is aimed at. You may also want to involve colleagues who will help to keep the blog going by posting regularly. You will then need to choose your blogging platform; either WordPress, Blogger or Medium are good places to start as they are free and relatively easy to get started.

Rather than creating your own blog, you may choose to signpost participants to links to other blogs where people have shared their experiences of living with, for example, diabetes.

Microblogs

Like blogs, microblogs can be used to keep group education participants informed about your education sessions or to disseminate news and updates related to the subject area. Twitter is the most popular microblog and has a 140-character limit meaning that you need to keep posts short and to the point. Using hashtags does mean that you are able to create a thread or discussion if this is the intention. Other examples of microblogs include Tumblr and Pinterest.

For a more detailed review of the use of social media in healthcare you can read: Grajales *et al.* (2014).

> ## TOP TIPS FOR USING THE INTERNET AND TEACHING ONLINE
>
> - Online material needs to be kept current therefore you will need to think about when the information should be updated or removed from the website.
> - Check URL links regularly to make sure they still connect to the appropriate web page.
> - To set up a social networking or blog account you will need to link it to an email address. Where possible use a generic organizational email rather than an individual one. This means that if you are off work or leave the organization, the account can still be accessed.
> - Keep professional and personal internet accounts separate.
> - Regularly monitor discussion forums and social networking sites so that you can respond promptly to questions and address any issues of inappropriate content.
> - Particularly when using discussion forums and social networking sites make sure that the ground rules are clear. They should provide guidance on how participants should interact online, for example, participants should be courteous and refrain from personal abuse; the forum should only be used for discussion related to the subject area and not for spam; it is also important, depending on the privacy settings of the site, to remind participants that their posts will be publicly available.

Online group education

Technology now allows you to develop group education sessions that are delivered online. If you have attended or worked in a higher education institute in the last 10–15 years, you are likely to have encountered a virtual learning environment (VLE) such as Blackboard, Moodle or WebCT. VLEs provide a platform upon which you can build an interactive online course that includes self-directed learning tasks for participants to engage with, discussion boards and group activities that can be worked on collaboratively. In addition to the VLE, web conferencing software such as Adobe Connect, Collaborate and WebX is available that allows you to create a virtual classroom where you can facilitate your group education session.

TOP TIP FOR LEARNING MORE ABOUT ONLINE EDUCATION

If you are interested in online education but don't have any experience of learning online, sign up to do a Massive Open Online Course (MOOC). MOOCs are free and available in many different subject areas. Coursera and FutureLearn are the main learning platforms which, in collaboration with global universities and organizations, offer a diverse catalogue of free online courses. Alternatively, you could join a live webinar to see how they work. This personal insight will give you some ideas of how online group education could work.

For those of you that are not associated with an organization that holds licenses for a server-based VLE and web conferencing software, there are other options. Coursesites by Blackboard is hosted in a web browser so it doesn't need a computer server or a license. It also integrates well with a free version of Collaborate so that you can hold webinars. An alternative is to use Google apps to create a Google site and use Google hangouts to set up a webinar. Skype also allows group video calls recommended for up to five people.

Here are **three basic considerations** if you are thinking about setting up an online education session:

1 **Support**: Do you have the support from a learning technologist or IT specialist? If you are planning an online education session it is essential to include them as part of the team. Learning technologists understand the practical issues of what will and won't work in the VLE, alongside the pedagogy of online learning. If you are holding webinars they will also be experienced at troubleshooting connection problems during the session, so inviting them to co-facilitate is a good idea.

2 **Access**: Will your target audience have internet access and the technological ability and confidence to interact online? For example, when using web conferencing software participants usually need to create an account, this in itself can create a barrier for people who are not confident online. Ideally, they will also need to have a webcam, and certainly an audio headset, so that they can take part in the session. Mobile apps are available for the majority of the VLEs and webinar tools and this may be something that participants can take advantage of.

3 **Content**: How will you structure the session and what will you include? Generally speaking, the principles of how to plan, deliver and evaluate an online session remain the same as when you are delivering it face-to-face. One difference that you will need to consider is if you want to include 'asynchronous' group activities that can be done by individual participants

in their own time such as watching a video then commenting on a discussion board or synchronous 'live' sessions such as a group webinar. You may of course choose a combination of the two.

As the twenty-first century progresses, undoubtedly our use of technology will increase further. Alongside this, the expectations of healthcare providers and users are likely to include more flexible access to healthcare education. For some members of the community and healthcare workers, education sessions delivered online offer this opportunity. Group members can participate with online sessions without leaving their home or place of work. This is an advantage in terms of reducing travel time and associated costs for participants and facilitators. For people that have problems accessing transport or childcare, or for those who are housebound, online learning offers the potential to reach individuals who may previously have been excluded from taking part in group education.

5.4 Ending a session

Evaluation is an essential part of delivering an education session and this will be considered in detail in Chapter 7. At the end of session, in addition to evaluation, you may also choose to include an activity that encourages self-reflection and reinforces action planning. This may include asking participants to spend a few minutes writing down their main learning points and, where appropriate, what they intend to do differently. You may wish to ask participants to identify, for example, one key learning point or an 'Ah-ha!' moment from the session, that they can feedback to the group.

It is important to finish a session on time as many participants will need to leave promptly and the room may be needed for other activities. Make sure that participants are clear about what happens next. In some cases, the session is a one off and there are no plans to see participants again, but with a series of sessions participants need to be clear when and where the next session will be, particularly if it is to be at a different venue. Facilitators may want to provide their contact details so that participants can contact them; they may recommend that participants undertake specific activities prior to the next session. All of this needs to be clearly explained. Clearing away resources can also take time and often participants will want to talk further to the facilitator. Facilitators should reflect on the session and make notes about how it went from their perspective. It is easy to forget if this is not done at the time. Thinking about what went well, what could have been better and recording any ideas of what could be done differently next time is a very useful activity.

References

Grajales III FJ, Sheps S, Ho K, Novak-Lauscher H and Eysenbach G (2014). Social media: a review and tutorial of applications in medicine and health care. *J Med Internet Res* 16(2): e13.

Exley K (2010). Encouraging active learning in lectures. *The All Ireland Journal of Teaching and Learning in Higher Education* 2(1): 10.1–10. [Online]. Available at http://ojs.aishe.org/index.php/aishe-j/article/view/10/14 [Accessed May 2016].

Eysenbach G (2001). What is e-health? *J Med Internet Res* 3(2): e20.

Internet Statistics Live (2015). Number of internet users [Online]. Available from: www.internetlivestats.com/ [Accessed May 2016].

Lal S and Adair C (2014). E-mental health: A rapid review of the literature. *Psychiat Serv* 65(1): 24–32.

Pal K, Eastwood SV, Michie S, Farmer A, Barnard ML *et al.* (2014). Computer-based interventions to improve self-management in adults with type 2 diabetes: a systematic review and meta-analysis. *Diabetes Care* 37(6): 1759–1766.

Further reading

Exley K and Dennick R (2004). *Small Group Teaching, Seminars and Beyond*. London: RoutledgeFalmer.

Grajales III FJ, Sheps S, Ho K, Novak-Lauscher H and Eysenbach G (2014). Social media: A review and tutorial of applications in medicine and health care *J Med Internet Res* 16(2): e13.

Useful websites

www.coursera.org/about/partners
www.futurelearn.com/courses/categories

Chapter 6 **Resources**

Vanessa Halliday

6.1 Introduction

The resources that you use are an important part of your education session. They should be designed and implemented in a way that will help the participants to actively engage in the session and promote lifestyle change. There are many resources to choose from. Some, such as information booklets, will help participants to develop their knowledge and understanding whilst others may be designed with the aim of improving coping and self-management strategies, developing skills or challenging attitudes and beliefs. This chapter includes information on how to select inclusive educational resources. It goes on to give an overview of the types of resources that are available as well as examples of where they can be obtained from. It will also provide tips and consider copyright law, for those of you wishing to develop your own resources.

In addition to the educational resources that you will be using, the following list includes items that may be of practical use during the education session. Check to see which are available at the venue and which you need to take with you:

- Flip chart paper
- Flip chart marker pens
- Reusable adhesive such as sticky tack
- Pens and pencils for participants to use
- Whiteboard pens
- Whiteboard cleaning cloth
- Scissors
- Laptop
- Portable projector

How to Facilitate Lifestyle Change: Applying Group Education in Healthcare, First Edition.
Amanda Avery, Kirsten Whitehead and Vanessa Halliday.
© 2017 John Wiley & Sons, Ltd. Published 2017 by John Wiley & Sons, Ltd.

- Extension lead
- Wireless presentation slide changer
- Laser pointer
- Spare blank paper
- Post-it notes
- Participant register
- Participant name badges
- Spare copies of all resources.

6.2 Resources for inclusive education

If your aim is to encourage active engagement by all members of the group, using resources that will lead to inclusive participation is essential. This will help you to develop an environment where participants feel comfortable and valued. Understanding the key characteristics of your audience will help you to do this. Contacting participants in advance of the session is a good idea so that you have information about any specific learning needs as a result of, for example, mobility, visual or hearing impairments. In order to deliver inclusive education, the factors in Table 6.1 should be taken into account when planning which resources you will use.

6.3 Practical considerations when selecting which resources to use

In addition to making sure that the resources you choose are appropriate for the group, there are a number of practical factors that should be considered. First and foremost, the venue and facilities will dictate what resources you can use. For example, including presentation slides or a video will only be possible if there is a computer and screen in the room where the session will be held. Alternatively, it may be possible if you have access to portable equipment, to take this with you to the venue. Using web-based resources will also mean that you need to make sure that there is a reliable internet connection. If you are planning to use resources such as games or food mats you will need to check that the size of the room allows for this. The number of participants will also need to be considered, particularly in the context of whether you have enough copies or versions of the resource to be shared around the group.

Some resources, as will be discussed later, are available free of charge but for others there may be an associated cost. What budget you have for the session may influence your decisions. If it is the first time that the session has run and you are ordering new resources, you will also need to take into

Table 6.1 What to consider when selecting resources for inclusive education.

Points to consider	Questions to ask
Age	• Will group participants all be of a similar age? If not, are the resources appropriate for a generation diverse audience? • Particularly when educating children, are the resources age appropriate?
Gender	• Do the resources include, for example, case studies of the appropriate gender mix?
Culture	• Which is the most appropriate language for the resources to be written in? • Are the resources being used, for example, food models, representative of the culturally diverse diets of the participants? • Could the resources being used be perceived as being culturally insensitive in any way?
Mobility and dexterity	• Do any of the resources rely on the participants having a certain level of mobility or manual dexterity?
Visual impairment	• Is the text on the written resources clear and large enough (e.g. 12+ size sans serif font)? • Is the text on the presentation slides clear and large enough (e.g. 28+ sans serif font)?
Hearing impairment	• Has the presenter checked that participants can hear them, each other and the media resources? • Does the presenter need to project their voice and speak louder? • Is it possible to use videos with subtitles? • Is the presenter facing the audience when speaking so that participants can lip read if necessary?
Cognition and attention deficit	• Does the complexity of any of the resources rely on participants having a high level of cognition? • Could the duration of any of the activities mean that those with attention deficit disengage?
Literacy level	• Is the language being used at the appropriate level and avoiding the use of unfamiliar abbreviations and jargon? • Do written resources follow the principles set out by, for example, the **Plain English Campaign**?
Digital literacy	• Are all participants likely to be familiar with the technology that they are being asked to use? • Will all participants have internet access? If not, have alternative sources of information been provided?
Specific learning difficulties, for example dyslexia	• Have written and verbal instructions for the activities been provided that are clear and well structured? • Have participants been provided with written materials in advance so that they can use their own coping strategies to prepare for the session?

account how long the delivery time is and if the resources will arrive in time. Availability may also need to be factored in if you are using resources that are on loan and need to be booked in advance.

6.4 Types of resources

There are many different types of resources available for you to use. Generally speaking, they should look professional, be interesting, affordable and where relevant, durable.

Written paper-based resources

Most educational sessions will include written paper-based resources that the participants will take away with them. In some cases, these will be professionally printed booklets and leaflets and in others, it may be necessary for you to write and print them yourself.

As with all resources, you will need to decide when is the most appropriate time in the session to hand them out to participants. For example, giving all of the paper-based resources out at the start is important if you expect participants to refer to the content as the session progresses. It also means that participants can make notes as you go along. However, depending on the number of resources you are using it may mean that there are numerous leaflets and sheets of paper for participants to manage. If you decide to wait until the end of the session make sure participants are aware of this so that they know that they will have the relevant information to take home with them.

TOP TIP WHEN USING MULTIPLE PAPER-BASED RESOURCES

Rather than printing all of the session information and resources on white A4 paper, use different coloured pastel shades of papers. For example, print the programme for the day on light blue paper and any quizzes on pale yellow paper. This way it is easier for you to find and refer to each of the hand-outs and for participants to identify which one you are talking about.

Developing your own written resources

There are a number of stages to consider when developing your own resources.

Before you begin

- Developing and printing your own resources takes time and energy so, rather than reinventing the wheel, check with colleagues and on the internet to see if there is already something available that you can use.

- Some organizations have a standard recommended template and process for developing printed materials that you may need to follow.
- Set yourself a realistic time frame. Particularly if you intend to collaborate with others and outsource the printing, this will be several weeks rather than days.

Writing the resource
- Review the relevant research literature so that you are confident that you are giving up-to-date evidence based advice.
- Consider the size and layout. Use headings and subheadings, avoid too much text on one page and leave space between paragraphs. Where relevant, include appropriately labelled diagrams and pictures.
- Use an easy to read sans serif font such as Arial or Verdana, point size 12 to 14 and justify the text to the left. Generally speaking, dark text on a light background is most legible.
- Write the first draft of the document including a brief introduction, aim of the resource, who it is for, key messages and summary.
- Avoid using abbreviations and jargon and where necessary, explain complex terms. If your resources are to be written in English, following the guidance from The Plain English Campaign should help to ensure that they are easy to read.
- Contact details that should be included on the resource are a telephone number, postal and email address. If you choose to include a contact name be aware that it may limit the resources shelf-life if there is a change in staffing.
- Relevant logos, organizations, department names and websites, as well as the date the information was produced and copyright information should also be included.
- Proof read the draft document.

Reviewing and editing
- It is good practice to send a draft version to colleagues and, where relevant, patient groups for their input. Be clear about what you would like comments on as well as the deadline by which they should respond.
- Make any final amendments.
- Proof read the final version.

Printing
- Decide on how you will print the resource. Using an external company will no doubt cost more money but should give you a more professional finish.
- Usually printing is more cost effective if you are ordering large volumes, however, you will need to bear in mind that the resource may become outdated. Using fewer colours can help to keep down the cost.

- Alternatively, you may choose to print the resource yourself. Particularly if photocopying, check to make sure that it is of suitable print quality and each side of the document has printed correctly in sequence.
- Printing on both sides of the page will save paper and money. Be mindful that if you do this and the quality of the paper is poor, the text may be visible on both sides of the page and could be illegible.

Slide presentations

Tips on how to format and structure presentation slides were discussed in Chapter 5. You may choose to print out a copy of the slides for participants to write notes on and take home. If this is the case, there are several points to consider.

- Decide how many slides to print on each page. For example, three slides positioned vertically, to the left of each page, should mean that the text is large enough to be read with space for participants to write notes next to each slide.
- Check to see that the printed slides are legible. This is particularly important if you have used smaller or light coloured font.
- If you are doing group work you may choose to omit some of the presentation slides from the printed copy, particularly if they contain the 'answers' to a question that you have asked. If this is the case, leaving a blank slide in the printed version means that participants are able to note down any relevant information that is discussed.

Using flip charts and white boards

Flip charts and whiteboards are useful resources that can support active participant engagement in the session. The following points can help you to use them effectively:

- Make sure all participants can see the white board and/or flip chart.
- Check that you have the correct paper for the flip chart. If not, anchoring the paper in place will be tricky.
- Use a non-permanent, dry erase marker pen for the white board. Permanent marker pens work better on paper. Blue and black ink are usually easier to read.
- Consider drawing more complex diagrams or pictures in advance of the session starting.
- Write legibly, large enough for people to read from a distance.
- If you are unsure how to spell a word, ask the audience rather than spelling it incorrectly.

Lay experts

In Chapter 1, we highlighted how lay and peer-led group education can be used to facilitate lifestyle change. An alternative to this approach is to involve someone that has personal experience of the subject area in the session that you are facilitating. For example, a weight management session could involve someone that has successfully lost weight talking about their experience, the challenges and how their life has changed as a consequence. Identifying an appropriate individual is important as some people may not feel comfortable discussing their experiences within a group setting whilst others may not be confident with public speaking. The organization that you work for may have contact details for laypeople that would like to be involved in education. Alternatively, local community or support groups might be able to put you in touch with volunteers.

Discussing expectations prior to getting final agreement from them that they are happy take part, is important. This should include, for example, if they will be paid for their time and, the very least, travel expenses should be offered. Being clear about the aim of their involvement, along with what they will focus on and include, will help to ensure that their participation is a positive experience for them, as well as being well received by the audience. A debrief after the session has ended will help you to gauge how they felt the session went and importantly, if they would like to be involved again in the future.

Additional resources

There are many examples of additional resources that are available. Some will need to be purchased, whereas others will be available on loan or free to use from the internet. Table 6.2 includes ideas of resources that you can use along with examples of where then can be obtained from. At the end of this chapter are four case studies that you can work through that will give you more ideas and information about resources that are relevant to; (1) alcohol awareness, (2) healthy eating, (3) physical activity and (4) smoking cessation.

6.5 General considerations when using resources

Used effectively resources can make the education session interesting and interactive. To make sure that the session is memorable for the right reasons you need to be familiar with the resources that you are using. Practice and pilot games, watch and listen to any multimedia resources that you will be using, read through written information and importantly, know how the technology works.

Table 6.2 Resource ideas and availability.

Resource ideas	Examples of where resources can be obtained from
Visual aids Anatomical models, e.g. the heart, the consequences of obesity, smoking, alcohol BMI calculators Children's stickers, badges and picture cards Fat vest Food items, packets and labels Food models Menu plans Posters The Eatwell Plate floor mat	Change4Life www.nhs.uk/change4life/ comic company www.comiccompany.co.uk/ Health Edco www.healthedco.co.uk/ Intimex www.eintimex.org Vitamex Nutricion www.vitamexdeoccidente.com/
Multimedia Audio recordings Film/TV programme clips Health related DVDs Magazine articles Newspaper articles Patient education videos Patient stories Photographs	YouTube www.youtube.com Patient education videos American College of Physicians www.acponline.org/patients_families/products/watch_videos/ NHS Choices www.nhs.uk Diabetes Stories produced by Oxford Centre for Diabetes, Endocrinology and Metabolism (OCDEM) www.diabetes-stories.com/
Games Food portion sizes Reading food labels Guess the food group Rate the fat, sugar, salt How much is a unit of alcohol? How to burn 100 calories Children's games such as snakes and ladders, card match, jigsaws, stamps and stickers	comic company www.comiccompany.co.uk/ Medline Interactive Health Games www.nlm.nih.gov/medlineplus/games.html Playnormous www.playnormous.com/
Other sources of educational resources Booklets Generic teaching materials Leaflets Self-assessment questionnaires	Health related charities, for example: American Heart Association www.my.americanheart.org/professional/Library/Library_UCM_316893_LibraryPage.jsp British Nutrition Foundation Resources

(Continued)

Table 6.2 (Continued)

Resource ideas	Examples of where resources can be obtained from
	www.nutrition.org.uk/foodinschools/ teachercentre/resources
	The British Heart Foundation www.bhf.org.uk/publications
	Local Government Organizations, Ministries of Health and Health Promotion Boards, for example:
	Public Health England www.campaigns.dh.gov.uk/
	The Ministry of Health of Turkey, Public Health Institution www.beslenme.gov.tr
	Singapore Health Promotion Board www.hpb.gov.sg/HOPPortal/faces/Resources
	Portuguese Department of Public Health Program for healthy eating in Schools www.passe.com.pt/
	Generic teaching resources, for example: Pinterest www.pinterest.com/
	TES resources www.tes.co.uk/teaching-resources

Time management

Whatever the size and dynamic of the group, using resources often takes longer than you think. Allow enough time to ensure that participants get the most out of the activity. Observe the group closely to ensure that participants haven't finished early and are becoming disengaged.

Health and safety

Resources should meet the required safety standards in term of, for example, manufacturing and materials. This, along with choosing age-appropriate resources, is particularly important when educating children. You may also need to consider where relevant, electrical testing of equipment that you are using. If your education session involves participants eating food, attention should be given to food safety and hygiene regulations.

Copyright

Copyright (symbol © or ℗ for a sound recording) is the legal protection given to the creator of an original piece of work, for example, text, video, art or music. Copyright law prevents the work from being copied, adapted or shared, unless the permission of the creator has been granted. If you choose to develop your own educational resources, the copyright will belong to you and 'all rights will be reserved' meaning that it cannot be copied, amended or re-used without your permission (GOV.UK, 2016). The majority of countries in the world are signed up to the Berne Convention which means that copyright is automatic and not something that you have to apply for. If you wish for your work to be made publicly available, and free to share, you may wish to attribute copyright permissions through a Creative Commons license and upload it to an appropriate open education resources internet site.

When developing your own resources, you should be mindful of making sure that you do not infringe copyright law by inadvertently using materials or images without the permission of the creator and/or without the correct acknowledgement or attribution. It is important to consider that, although many of the underpinning principles are the same, copyright law can differ between countries. Recent changes in the UK mean that there are certain exceptions to the law when the material is being used for educational purposes. To read more about this you can access the GOV.UK website and the Exceptions to copyright: Education and Teaching (2014) document produced by the Intellectual Property Office.

Creative Commons licenses

Creative Commons is a non-profit organization that has developed a standardized range of free-to-use licenses and tools that allow you, as the creator of a resource, the ability to grant copyright permissions. There are a number of licenses available that provide a range of options related to the level at which you wish for your resource to be copied, adapted or shared. For example, the Attribution (CC BY) license allows others to distribute, amend and re-share your work providing they acknowledge you as the original creator. This includes use for commercial purposes. The Attribution-ShareAlike (CC BY-SA) license allows the same, but has an additional stipulation that any new resources that are created from the original must be licensed under the same terms. Other licenses, such as the Attribution-NoDerivs (CC BY-ND), do not allow for any changes to the original work to made, but do allow for re-distribution providing the correct acknowledgements are in place.

You can read more about Creative Commons licenses at https:// creativecommons.org/licenses/.

Open education resources

Open educational resources (OERs) are educational materials that are freely available online for anyone to use. They have an open-license which means that you are legally able to copy, edit, add to them and re-share as you require.

The range of OERs is diverse and includes videos, photographs, images and presentation slides as well as entire university course materials. They can be found on the internet at sites such as YouTube, i-Tunes U, SlideShare and OER Commons. Many educational institutions and organizations such as MIT OpenCourseWare will also have OERs. In Brazil, for example, all educational materials that are produced with public money are open-licensed. To read more about OERs you can access 'A guide to open educational resources' on the Jisc website.

Most OERs will have a Creative Commons license that will tell you exactly how you can use and reuse the resource. Or, in the case of free software, it is likely to be a GNU General Public License.

6.6 Case studies

Consider the following scenarios with regards to the resources that you would use. Discussion of the approach that the facilitator could take, along with examples of resources, is given next:

Case study 6.1 Alcohol awareness

Educating students about the dangers of binge drinking has been identified as a local priority. As such, your organization has been commissioned to deliver a 1-hour education session in 10 of the local higher education colleges.
- What factors should be considered when using resources with this group?
- What resources could you use in these sessions?

FACILITATOR APPROACH TO ALCOHOL AWARENESS RESOURCES

Given that the age range of the group is likely to be late teens or early twenties, it is likely that participants will have a high level of digital literacy. As such, using interactive technology within the session may help to stimulate their interest, participation and learning. For example, you could use audience response 'clicker' systems to collect responses to questions from the group or online interactive quizzes that individuals can complete during the session. Involving a 'lay expert' who can talk about their experience and negative consequences of binge drinking would be a powerful way of getting important messages over to the group.

Consideration should be given to the fact that there may be some members of the group that are under the legal drinking age, or are from cultural backgrounds where alcohol is prohibited. Particularly if you are planning on providing resources to be taken away at the end of the session, it is important to consider how these will be received by the students' family members.

As you will be delivering the session ten times in different locations you will need to consider the cost, availability and portability of any technology and other resources that you use.

Ideas for resources and where they can be obtained from include:

The Drinkaware website, www.resources.drinkaware.co.uk/, includes an extensive range of resources including an online unit calculator and assess your drinking activity. There are also a number of free to download factsheets including 'Alcohol and Young People'. Additional resources that are available to purchase include unit and calorie calculators, unit measure cups and an interactive alcohol fact or fiction quiz for children to learn about the risks of underage drinking.

The Change4Life website, www.nhs.uk/Change4Life/Pages/drink-less-alcohol. aspx, includes an online interactive drinks checker and alcohol tracker mobile app.

The NHS publication, 'Your drinking and you: The facts on alcohol and how to cut down', www.alcohollearningcentre.org.uk/_library/Change4Life/408723_ Your_Drinking_And_You.pdf, is a comprehensive printed booklet that includes information about alcohol and the health risks, behaviour change self-assessment questionnaires and goal setting activities.

Public Health England, www.alcohollearningcentre.org.uk/, have a range of alcohol learning resources including an e-learning course for professional who will be delivering alcohol awareness education.

Case study 6.2 Healthy eating

You have been asked to do a 2-hour (9.30–11.30 am) education session in the local school to a group of 5–8 year olds. The topic is 'Fruit and Vegetables'.

• What factors should be considered when using resources with this group?
• What resources could you use in this session?

FACILITATOR APPROACH TO HEALTHY EATING RESOURCES

Some of the children, particularly the younger ones, are likely to have short attention spans. For this reason, including activities that use resources that are interactive is important. Games such as bingo or card match can be fun as well as educational, with stickers as rewards for those that take part.

Using food models or photographs can help children to identify fruit and vegetables, Alternatively, including 'real' fruit and vegetables will provide an opportunity for the children to feel and smell items that they may be unfamiliar with. The timing of the session also means that there will be a mid-morning break when you could get the children to try fruit and vegetable snacks.

Ideas for resources and where they can be obtained from include:

The comic company, www.comiccompany.co.uk/, have 'Eat 5' jigsaws and bingo games that are available to purchase. They also have a range of fruit and vegetable stickers.

The TES website, www.tes.co.uk/teaching-resources, includes many fruit and vegetable related ideas and resources including colouring in pages, fruit multiplication and flashcards.

Short video clips and songs, such as the Barnaby Bear 'Five a Day' song on the BBC education website, www.bbc.co.uk/education/clips/z2pxpv4, can be included in the session by getting the children to sing along.

Case study 6.3 Physical activity

The local Rural and Community Action Group has recently been focussing its work on promoting physical activity in older people. You have agreed to facilitate a series of six hour long sessions that will be held weekly in the village hall. The sessions are aimed at the over 65-year age group.

• What factors should be considered when using resources with this group?

• What resources could you use in this session?

FACILITATOR APPROACH TO PHYSICAL ACTIVITY RESOURCES

Particularly as this is a series of six sessions, it is likely that you will want to include practical activities that get the participants moving. If this is the case, you may need to take with you exercise mats and other exercise equipment such as dumbbells or weights. The practicalities of transporting this and whether it can be stored at the venue will need to be considered. Likewise, if you are planning on doing, for example, seated exercises, you will need to check that the chairs in the venue are appropriate. For these types of activities, it is important that the participants have the correct type of footwear and clothing. Information about this should be included in the pre-course information. You may choose to set between-session activities using pedometers. Although pedometers can be purchased relatively cheaply their use, along with the other exercise equipment, may well be dictated by the size of your budget.

An important consideration for this type of session is that the activities you include are appropriate for the level of fitness of the group. The BHF National Centre website, www.bhfactive.org.uk/older-adults/index.html, includes some useful resources for people that are planning physical activity education sessions for older adults. The National Institute on Aging website, www.nia.nih.gov/health/publication/exercise-physical-activity/introduction, also has available an e-guide for exercise and physical activity that includes sample exercises for endurance, balance, strength and flexibility.

Case study 6.4 Smoking cessation

The cardiac rehabilitation programme that is organized and run by the local hospital includes a 90-minute session on smoking cessation. The hospital is in an inner city area that has an ethnically diverse population. The previous facilitator has recently left and you have agreed to deliver the session that runs once every 8 weeks.

• What factors should be considered when using resources with this group?
• What resources could you use in this session?

FACILITATOR APPROACH TO SMOKING CESSATION RESOURCES

Given the location of the hospital it is likely that the participants attending this group will be from different ethnic backgrounds. It is therefore important to use resources that represent the cultural diversity of the group, particularly with regards to how tobacco products are used.

Demonstrating how smoking and tobacco can damage the body using an anatomical model is one way for participants to understand the health risks.

Models, however, can be expensive to buy but, as this is an ongoing education programme, you may decide that the cost is warranted. An alternative is to show what can happen in the body using diagrams or pictures. Involving an expert patient in the session who can discuss their own experiences of stopping smoking, is something that participants should be able to relate to. Ideas for resources and where they can be obtained from include:

The Quit website, www.quit.org.uk/, includes many resources such as a Smoking quiz, behaviour change self-assessment questionnaire 'Your quit plan' and booklets that can be ordered, for example, 'So you want to quit?'

The NHS Smokefree resources, www.nhs.uk/smokefree, include an 'Addiction test' and videos of 'Success stories'.

Action on Smoking and Health (ASH), www.ash.org.uk/, and Centers for Disease Control and Prevention (CDC), www.cdc.gov/tobacco/index.htm, websites both contain a wealth of information and resources such as multimedia campaigns, presentation slides and links to YouTube videos.

References

GOV.UK (2016) How copyright protects your work [Online] Available from: www.gov.uk/copyright [Accessed May 2016].

Intellectual Property Office (2014). Exceptions to copyright: Education and Teaching [Online] Available from: www.gov.uk/government/uploads/system/uploads/attachment_data/file/375951/Education_and_Teaching.pdf [Accessed May 2016].

Useful websites

American College of Physicians www.acponline.org/patients_families/products/watch_videos/

American Heart Association www.my.americanheart.org/professional/Library/Library_UCM_316893_LibraryPage.jsp

Action on Smoking and Health (ASH) www.ash.org.uk/

BBC Education www.bbc.co.uk/education

British Heart Foundation www.bhf.org.uk/publications

British Nutrition Foundation Resources www.nutrition.org.uk/foodinschools/teachercentre/resources

Centers for disease control and prevention www.cdc.gov

Change4Life www.nhs.uk/change4life/

comic company www.comiccompany.co.uk/

Creative commons www.creativecommons.org/licenses/

Diabetes Stories produced by Oxford Centre for Diabetes, Endocrinology and Metabolism (OCDEM) www.diabetes-stories.com/

Drinkaware website www.resources.drinkaware.co.uk/

Health Edco www.healthedco.co.uk/
Intimex www.eintimex.org
JISC digital technology www.jisc.ac.uk/
Medline Interactive Health Games www.nlm.nih.gov/medlineplus/games.html
Ministry of Health of Turkey, Public Health Institution www.beslenme.gov.tr
NHS Choices www.nhs.uk
NHS Smokefree www.nhs.uk/smokefree
Pinterest www.pinterest.com/
Playnormous www.playnormous.com/
Plain English campaign www.plainenglish.co.uk/
Portuguese Department of Public Health Program for healthy eating in Schools www.passe.com.pt/
Public Health England www.campaigns.dh.gov.uk/
Quit www.quit.org.uk
Singapore Health Promotion Board www.hpb.gov.sg/HOPPortal/faces/Resources
TES resources www.tes.co.uk/teaching-resources
Vitamex Nutricion www.vitamexdeoccidente.com/
YouTube www.youtube.com

Chapter 7 **Evaluation**

Kirsten Whitehead

7.1 Introduction

Evaluation is a key part of developing effective group education. It can easily become something of an afterthought, but should be planned in advance and linked to the objectives and learning outcomes of the session.

This chapter begins by looking at the theoretical understanding of what evaluation is in the context of group education, why evaluation is undertaken (and the benefits of it), what exactly should be evaluated and who might complete the evaluation.

The chapter then moves on to look more practically at what methods could be used and what needs to be considered in order to meet the needs of group members. Cases and examples are included to support the reader to think through the practicalities.

7.2 What is evaluation?

Evaluation has been described by Rootman *et al.* (2001) as the systematic examination and assessment of features of a programme or other intervention in order to produce knowledge that different stakeholders can use for a variety of purposes. Evaluation is about judging the value of an activity and assessing whether or not it has achieved what it set out to do (Cavill *et al.*, 2015). Evaluation in the context of group education can provide information about the extent to which the session (or group of sessions) met its aim and objectives and whether participants achieved the learning outcomes. It should not be seen as a complex process but a normal part of everyday education practice; if an education session is delivered, it is evaluated. Questions such as 'Is the right content being delivered? and 'Is it working?' will be relevant.

How to Facilitate Lifestyle Change: Applying Group Education in Healthcare, First Edition.
Amanda Avery, Kirsten Whitehead and Vanessa Halliday.
© 2017 John Wiley & Sons, Ltd. Published 2017 by John Wiley & Sons, Ltd.

7.3 Why evaluate?

The value to stakeholders is both from the point of view of the consequences of the session (does it work?) but also the costs of the investment of time, money, knowledge and skills of facilitators and resources required. Financial resources are increasingly scarce and economic (or fiscal) evaluation can address the costs and benefits of the investment. Economic evaluation is defined as the comparative analysis of alternative courses of action in terms of both their costs and consequences (Drummond et al., 2005). Full economic evaluation requires highly skilled personnel to undertake it and will not be used for every project or intervention, but all facilitators and their managers should be concerned about the cost-effectiveness of the education being undertaken. Is it a good use of resource? Could the same results be achieved with a smaller outlay of resource? Evaluation itself uses resources and can be costly so a clear purpose for it is essential (Naidoo and Wills, 2009). Group education has taken the place of one to one consultations in some instances as it is thought to be more cost-effective but that is only true if the session is well delivered and meets the learning needs of the participants.

Cost is important but evaluation has many other benefits. Table 7.1 gives a variety of reasons for, and benefits of, evaluation, with examples related to delivering group education. The priorities for 'why' evaluation is undertaken will influence 'what' is evaluated and 'how' it is completed. Evaluation itself is only going to be worthwhile if the facilitator acts on the results. If the group education is being delivered by a group of facilitators, then they all need to be 'on board' and willing to act on what the evaluation reveals.

7.4 What to evaluate?

It is important to consider exactly what sort of evaluation to conduct right from the beginning of the development of the group education (Cavill et al., 2015). The level of evaluation will vary and be more or less formal (Naidoo and Wills, 2009) depending on a variety of factors including the requirements of funders. In group education, both participants and facilitators views will be of interest. In many cases the facilitator will have to consider what is realistic. Full economic evaluation is costly and is not going to be necessary for a one-off group education session about healthy eating on a budget! The evaluation needs to be in proportion to the size and scale of the work being delivered and the resources for the evaluation incorporated.

There are different types of evaluation that are frequently considered and these relate to:

• Formative: part of the development process
• Process: the way things are done

Table 7.1 Reasons for undertaking evaluation.

Reason for evaluation	Example
To see what has been achieved	Although most of the achievements of a session will hopefully be related to the aim and objectives, sometimes there are unexpected achievements. Evaluation will help to identify these. An education session that has not demonstrated achievements cannot be considered effective (Holli *et al.*, 2014).
To help facilitators to reflect and improve practice	A good facilitator will always be looking for ways to improve what they do. Evaluation should not just be the participant's perspective but the facilitator should be asking themselves questions about how well the session went and if there is anything that can be changed to improve it. Participant feedback will aid this process.
To check if the objectives have been met or not	It is important to remember that although it is good if participants (and facilitator) enjoy a session, that is not the primary aim. The session must demonstrate that it is achieving the objectives it was designed to deliver.
To measure progress (against specified goals)	In some cases, a service will have been commissioned to deliver a session or series of session within a time frame. Continuous evaluation will demonstrate if appropriate progress towards those goals is being made.
To identify strengths and weaknesses	Even with well-planned sessions it is likely that there will be some aspects of the session that could be improved. An activity planned to deliver a specific learning outcome may not work as well as hoped and may need to be replaced by a different activity or adjusted in some way. Identifying weaknesses allows the facilitator to direct their work to the areas most in need of adjustment.
To see if anything is going wrong and to ensure you are doing no harm!	Some facilitators may assume that their good intentions will work well for participants and lead to a positive outcome. However, it is important to look out for unexpected negative outcomes, for example has any participant been excluded in any way, has the facilitator (or other participants) judged an individual creating a barrier to behaviour change rather than a support?
To assess acceptability/ stakeholder satisfaction	It is essential that the session is acceptable to the participants and also those who have commissioned the service. For example, a session designed to promote a healthy diet would need to consider the dietary habits and income of the participants. If participants have dietary restrictions as part of the observance of their faith this should be considered in the way food is discussed. Similar considerations would need to be incorporated when discussing alcohol or appropriate types of physical activity. Not doing so is disrespectful and may alienate participants.

(Continued)

Table 7.1 (Continued)

Reason for evaluation	Example
To inform future plans	Evaluation allows future plans to take into account what has already happened and the learning from that. It may be that the facilitator has been able to identify other sessions or activities that would enhance the participants' experience and ability to change lifestyle behaviour. In effect there needs to be a feedforward mechanism so that this information can be used not just by that specific facilitator but also by others who may be delivering similar sessions.
To be able to share experiences	The need for lifestyle change is global and there will be many very similar sessions being delivered across the world. Sharing what has worked well and what didn't can help those developing sessions in a different geographical area. Comprehensive and well conducted evaluations can sometimes be published as abstracts or research papers. More commonly, a report or presentation will be prepared that can be shared across or within professions or organizations and be useful to others.
To secure funding	Locating funding to develop a new service is increasingly challenging. Often a thoroughly evaluated and costed pilot which provides evidence of effectiveness can be used to support the funding bid. Funders have to make very difficult decisions about where resource is directed and well evaluated services make their decisions more informed. Without evaluation it is very difficult to make a case for more resources or to expand a service (Naidoo and Wills, 2009).
To identify ways of improving monitoring methods	Evaluation can identify areas that are not being monitored, that should be, or help identify a better way to collect relevant data. What information might participants be willing and able to provide routinely to aid monitoring? Are they happy to be weighed, to keep records of steps taken using a pedometer, to keep food diaries and so on?
To make work more effective	Evaluating a session may help identify a simpler or more cost-effective activity to meet a learning outcome. The facilitator can then stop spending time on activities that do not help meet the objectives and develop more successful activities. A session can become more effective in relation to meeting its objectives as well as more cost-effective.
To develop theory	Although there is a lot of existing theory in relation to teaching and learning and behaviour change there are still unanswered questions. Evaluations can contribute to this knowledge and help develop it further. There is a drive to make healthcare services more evidence based and evaluation is part of that.

Table 7.1 (Continued)

Reason for evaluation	Example
To give a voice to the participants	Participants have a unique view of an education session and can identify strengths and weaknesses that a facilitator cannot. Participants may have had to take time off work or organize childcare, for example, to enable them to attend a session. They can be frustrated if they have spent time attending a session that was not useful, but having a means to give feedback can alleviate some of that frustration. Some may be very keen to support facilitators and have excellent suggestions for development.

- Impact: the immediate changes in knowledge, skills, behaviour, attitudes, belief or service use as a direct result of the group education session and
- Outcome: the effect or consequences of what is done that can be measured at various time points, short term or long term.

Formative evaluation

This refers to evaluation that takes place as part of the development process and guides the facilitator to develop an effective education programme for that target group (Cavill *et al.*, 2015). Sometimes this type of evaluation can be a formal research project, which then supplies pertinent information for facilitators. For example, Metzgar *et al.* (2014) utilized focus groups with women to identify facilitators and barriers to weight loss and weight loss maintenance. The information gained allows future interventions to address the issues identified. Similarly, Gillespie *et al.* (2014) identified triggers and barriers to parents and their children entering a childhood weight management service. Having completed the study, the authors were able to identify **who** parents wanted to deliver the service, **what** would appeal to them and **how** to recruit.

The following list is adapted from Cavill *et al.* (2015) and suggests a variety of approaches that can be included in formative evaluation:

- Undertaking needs assessment research
- Target group profiling: determining a detailed understanding of the relevant characteristics of the target group to allow the education to be tailored to their needs
- Pre-testing of materials: this can be really useful and many organizations, such as the UK NHS, provide guidance on producing information for patients, for example www.nhsidentity.nhs.uk/tools-and-resources/patient-information

- Piloting the session and then revising in light of evaluation
- Focus group discussions with potential target participants
- Informal discussions with target group participants
- Exploration of barriers and motivators to behaviour change
- Use of readability tests for resources to be used.

Although using formative evaluation can be time consuming and costly, it does increase the likelihood of the education session delivering its objectives and associated resources being well received. Facilitators may not necessarily need to undertake all of these approaches depending on what is known already about the needs of the target group and if existing resources are appropriate. Often formative evaluation informs the facilitator about the participants' ideas, opinions and values (Holli *et al.*, 2014).

Another description of formative evaluation is that which is undertaken as an education session is occurring and which allows the facilitator to assess learning during the education process. If participants appear unclear about an aspect of the learning the facilitator can then provide an alternative explanation that may help participants. In a future session the facilitator will be aware of the need to explain more clearly.

Process evaluation

This can be from the facilitator or participant perspective or from another stakeholder. It explores what is happening within the group education session and can be very helpful in providing explanations as to why objectives have or have not been met (Cavill *et al.*, 2015). It can also help with clarifying practicalities such as whether the session can be repeated, can be delivered in different settings or to similar groups of participants (Naidoo and Wills, 2009).

There are a range of questions that can be asked within a process evaluation. Table 7.2 lists these with some examples

Impact evaluation

This is what most facilitators will undertake routinely and it is usually relatively easy to do. It tends to be undertaken at the end of the session before participants leave. Some authors refer to this as the 'short-term outcome' (Cavill *et al.*, 2015). With impact evaluation, facilitators will be looking to see if short-term objectives and the participant learning outcomes have been achieved. These could be related to knowledge, skills, awareness or attitude.

Table 7.3 uses the lesson plan example from Chapter 4 to identify which objectives and learning outcomes are process evaluation and which are impact.

Table 7.2 Questions for process evaluation.

Question theme	Example
Reaching the target group	Are the people who are attending the people who the education session was designed for? If a session is designed to support healthy weight management then are the participants overweight or obese or carers of someone who is? If the session was designed to target at risk ethnic minority groups, is that who is attending? Are there enough participants from the target group attending to make it viable? A group education session can be very positively evaluated but if the numbers of participants attending are too small it will not be cost-effective to deliver.
Acceptability of the education session	Participants' satisfaction with a group education session is absolutely essential. Did they enjoy it? Was it useful? Was it appropriate for their needs? If the programme is not acceptable to participants the quality of the information provided becomes irrelevant. Participants are also less likely to come back or recommend the session to others. Participant views may vary depending on age, gender, ethnicity and other personal characteristics. Evaluating the acceptability of an education session therefore needs to be completed every time it is delivered to build a bigger picture than just the views of one group.
Practical arrangements	It is really important to check what participants thought of the venue and any refreshments. Were they suitable? For example, a statement like 'The venue provided an atmosphere conducive to learning' (i.e. space/temperature/facilities) with options to agree or disagree can be useful. Participants could rate refreshments from 0 to 5 where 0 was very poor and 5 was excellent. You may discover really useful information such as participants not being able to hear well due to noise from outside, that people were too cold (or hot) to concentrate or there was a mistake with directions. Uncomfortable surroundings can be a barrier to learning and paying attention to practical details is time well spent. Refreshments need to be suitable for all participants. This again will be important to consider particularly with participants from different ethnic backgrounds or with different faiths. It is good practice to ask about any specific needs that participants have in relation to food and drink prior to the session and to plan for these needs. Not considering such needs can be a barrier to building rapport with participants.
Delivering the plan	Did the facilitators actually deliver the education session as planned? If not, why not? Was there sufficient time? Was there enough material to fill the time? Did the planned activities work well? Sometimes activities work less well for very simple reasons such as a lack of table top or somewhere to put resources or a wall space. If participants are reluctant to participate in activities this can affect the time they take to complete.
Quality of the education	This relates not just to the material and activities delivered, but also the facilitator knowledge and skills. Resources used need to be up-to-date and appropriate for the participants. Facilitators need to be organized, managing time and group dynamics well. Did the content of the event meet participant expectations? Was the presentation of the subject clear and understandable?

Table 7.3 Linking process and impact evaluation to objectives and learning outcomes.

Objectives	Process or impact?
To inform participants of the current recommendations for physical activity	This is something the facilitator will know if they did or not and is therefore **process**.
To identify reasons for physical inactivity	This again is part of the **process**. The facilitator, if they have followed the lesson plan can tick this objective off as they know they did it with the participants.
To empower participants to plan realistic ways to increase their physical activity level	This is slightly more complicated as a facilitator cannot say 'yes I empowered the participants' without measuring the participants' perceptions of how empowered they are. They would therefore have to use some tool to measure this and it would be a part of the **impact**.
Learning Outcomes: By the end of the session, participants will:	

1. Be able to state four benefits of regular physical activity
 	
2. Have identified their current level of activity in relation to current recommendations
 	
3. Have identified at least one personal barrier to undertaking regular physical activity
 	
4. Be aware of at least three local services to access to increase activity
	These are all impact evaluation and will often be assessed by the verbal interaction with the group or by using a written questionnaire or quiz with direct questions such as:
	• Please state four benefits of regular physical activity
	• How would you rate your current levels of physical activity in relation to the current recommendations? (Please tick appropriate response):
	  ◦ I meet the recommendations fully
	  ◦ I nearly meet the recommendations
	  ◦ I do more than half the recommended amount of physical activity
	  ◦ I do less than half the recommended amount of physical activity
	• Please state one personal barrier to undertaking regular physical activity
	• Please state three local services that you could access to increase your physical activity level.

5. Have made an action plan of two things they will do over the next 2 weeks to increase their physical activity level	This is also an impact or short-term outcomes evaluation. Facilitators may have given time to do this within the group education session (i.e. completed the process) but whether participants have filled it in with appropriate actions is a different aspect of evaluation. This also relates back to the objective to 'To empower participants to plan realistic ways to increase their physical activity level'.

Outcome evaluation (long term)

Outcome evaluation is the focus on the long-term effect of the group education session and is far more difficult to measure than the short-term impact,
as well as requiring more resources (Naidoo and Wills, 2009). It assesses the
effectiveness of the group education against its objectives and is looking for a
sustained effect. Some education sessions will not have written long-term
objectives as they accept that they will not be able to measure them. It can
be a bit of a circular process and this is partly to do with access to the same
participants over a longer period of time. Will you be able to contact the
participants in 6 months and ascertain if they have improved their diet,
increased their physical activity level or decreased their body weight?
Sometimes this will be feasible and sometimes not. For example, it may be
possible to contact participants from a 6-week programme of cook and eat
education sessions after 6 months and ask them to report on dietary change.
Numbers may be relatively small and participants are likely to be local
making them more accessible. Ideally, a control group of people with similar
characteristics and needs but who had not attended the group education
would also be investigated to further evidence that it was the group education
specifically that had led to the change in behaviour.

Similar questions can be used as were asked for impact evaluation if
facilitators want to know if knowledge has been retained but there also needs
to be questions about behaviour change, assuming that was one of the aims
of the education.

Outcome evaluation has become easier with developments in information
technology and online surveys, particularly with staff groups, but the work
involved still has to be factored into the overall project costs. There is also a need
to have people with the skills to complete the statistical analysis and interpret the
results appropriately. Online surveys also allow for self-reported progress but
where objective measures of outcomes are required, such as weight loss or
change in blood pressure, then having a place for people to come to be measured, appropriate equipment and staff all need to be considered. Participants
will need to be contacted and appointments arranged, all of which is costly.

Although longer-term outcome evaluation can be undertaken it remains
difficult to link changes in behaviour with long-term health outcomes except
in large research studies with significant funding. In this case outcomes such
as mortality rates, evidence of negative health outcomes such as stroke or
myocardial infarction, or measurements such as Disability Adjusted Life
Years (DALYs) can be used.

Pragmatic evaluation involves selecting the most appropriate methods
according to the resources available and for group education this is
more likely to be the approach rather than using experimental or quasi-
experimental designs (Cavill *et al.*, 2015).

7.5 Who should evaluate?

Evaluation can be completed either by the facilitator themselves or by independent or external researchers and there are pros and cons to both.

Independent or external researchers

Independent or external researchers will add significant costs and are only likely to be used for bigger educational programmes. They are likely to take longer to understand the objectives of the project and establish contacts with participants. What participants say about an education programme may differ depending on who they are talking to. If they have built a good rapport with a facilitator, they may not feel able to criticize the education session to them but may feel better able to say what they really think to an independent person. However, they may feel more reserved with someone they do not know. Independent evaluators may be more objective and less biased than facilitators and are likely to have greater research expertise (Naidoo and Wills, 2009).

Facilitators themselves

Facilitators may have a better understanding of the education session, what can be improved and how, but may also be committed to self-justification and struggle to be objective. If evaluation has not been planned, costed and factored in to the time scale, other pressures can become an issue and evaluation may get pushed aside. However, this way of evaluation is likely to be the most cost-effective and realistic for most group education.

7.6 How to evaluate: tools and methods

Study design

There are several types of study design that can be used for evaluation, which include experimental designs, quasi-experimental designs, pre-experimental designs and post-intervention only. These are discussed in more detail by Cavill *et al.* (2015). An example of an experimental design is the formative evaluation, using a pilot randomized controlled trial, of the 'Waste the Waist' programme (Greaves *et al.*, 2015). This study measured recruitment and retention rates as well as weight loss and a range of blood biochemistry, dietary intake scores and physical activity measures. The results were compared between the participants who received the educational intervention and the control group who received usual care. Such a study provides the strongest level of evidence for the effectiveness of the education and is ideal if there are plans to roll out the programme across a larger geographical area and over a period of time. However, that is not the likely design of most educational sessions. Many will utilize pre-experimental designs that use pre-post intervention measures hoping to demonstrate impact. Whichever type of study design, there are a variety of measurement tools that can be used.

Evaluation methods and tools

Some evaluation tools collect purely qualitative data, some quantitative data and some are a combination of the two. Quantitative data may include how many people attended, measurements of weight, blood pressure, quality-of-life scores and so on. Qualitative data will give more depth and detail and help the facilitator understand **why** something does or does not work, which is really helpful when trying to decide on ways to improve the education session. Often a combination of both will be considered as they provide different information. Table 7.4 includes a summary of commonly used methods to consider and some of the advantages and disadvantages of their use.

Evaluation tools are often developed quickly with little thought about the questions and how they may be received. However, thoughtful design of a questionnaire, interview schedule or focus group topic guide is essential if the answers are going to be meaningful and answering the questions the facilitator really wants answered. Detailed guidance on preparing good quality surveys can be found in McColl *et al.* (2001), De Vaus (2002), De Leeuw *et al.* (2008) and Newell and Burnard (2011). In many cases, using more than one method of collating information will lead to a more comprehensive evaluation.

TOP TIPS FOR PREPARING EVALUATION QUESTIONNAIRES

- Take your time. It is not a 5-minute job.
- Make sure the language is clear.
- Think about response formats. Do you want to provide tick boxes or open text? The wording of the response formats is as important as the wording of the questions.
- Always give participants an opportunity to qualify what they are saying, for example please explain…
- Pre-test your questionnaire, get someone else to read it and ideally then pilot it on a group of participants with similar characteristics as the groups the questionnaire will be used for.
- Is the order of the questions logical?
- Make sure the instructions are clear. Should participants tick boxes, delete inappropriate responses, circle the right response? If they have to choose a number, for example 1 =poor, 5=excellent, make sure it is really clear which number relates to which response, as it is not unusual for people to get them the wrong way round.
- Questionnaires should look professional as this is known to increase the likelihood of people completing them (McColl *et al.*, 2001).
- Keep the questionnaire as short and simple as possible. Only ask questions that you really need to know the answer to.

Table 7.4 Evaluation methods.

Method	Examples	Considerations
Quantitative objective measures	Numbers of people attending session(s) or completing the whole course.	A very straightforward measure which should be routine. Sign-in sheets for participants will be a simple way to collect this. If attendance is poor for a session or attrition is high with a series of sessions this should raise concern.
	Body weight, blood pressure, blood biochemistry.	Require a trained person and appropriate equipment to ensure accurate measurements but are a good objective tool to measure if behaviour change has led to desired long-term outcomes or not.
	Step counts	Quality of pedometers is variable and results rely on the participant having used the pedometer correctly. There are many different tools now available that can be used, including those on mobile phones and other electronic devices.
	Participant data such as age and gender (to assess if the target group has been reached).	Usually available on referrals for patients or service users.
Individual interviews	Face-to-face, can be short and factual lasting only a few minutes, or longer using more exploratory questions (Bowling, 2009).	Can be affected by interviewer bias, i.e. the way the interviewer asks questions influences how the questions are answered. The relationship between the interviewer and the participant can affect the answers given. If the facilitator is the interviewer this will influence what the participant says. However, individual interviews can obtain really useful information about how a session has been received and why and how it could be developed. Interviews can also be affected by social desirability bias where participants say what they think will please the interviewer. If the interview(s) has/have been recorded they can be transcribed and analysed rigorously but this is more a research method and will not usually be undertaken without specific funding and a research protocol.

Table 7.4 (Continued)

Method	Examples	Considerations
	Telephone	Can be problems with people changing their telephone numbers frequently.
		Have you got permission to telephone the participant? If the evaluation is part of a research project, then you may be required to write to the participant to inform them that you are going to ring them. Alternatively, participants may sign consent forms during education sessions giving permission for them to be contacted for the purpose of service evaluation.
		Is the person on the phone who you think it is?
		Some people do not enjoy talking on the telephone and may purposely keep answers brief.
		The interviewer has no idea what is going on in the background which may be influencing the interview.
		Participants may have a hearing deficit which makes the interview more difficult.
		In theory a telephone interview is likely to be more cost effective than a face-to-face interview as it cuts down on travel costs.
		Telephone interviews are only really suitable for short questionnaires and it is easy for the participant to cut the interview short (Bowling, 2009).
Focus groups	Small groups of participants who interact with each other and the group leader	The key here is the interaction between the group leader and the participants that can stimulate discussion and generate ideas that may be different to one to one interviews.
		Focus groups can be undertaken with people who did attend but also those who did not (to ascertain why they did not attend).
		Participants can feel they are playing a positive and active part in the evaluation and development process.
		Managing a focus group requires similar skills to managing the group education session and all participants need to have a chance to contribute.
		A topic guide is needed to facilitate the discussion and ensure that the required subjects are covered.
		A comfortable environment needs to be provided.
		Some participants will find a focus group less intimidating than a one to one interview.

(Continued)

Table 7.4 (Continued)

Method	Examples	Considerations
Questionnaires	Paper questionnaires given out at the end of an education session	Participants may be in a hurry to leave and not consider their answers very fully or complete them at all. There is no interviewer bias. Some participants may have problems with literacy or language and therefore not complete the questionnaire. There are fewer problems with social desirability bias than with interviews.
	Postal questionnaires	Who actually completes the questionnaire? Can you be sure it is the participant? It is easy for participants to ignore these and not complete them for a variety of reasons. Response rates can be low. Requires correct addresses for participants.
	Electronic questionnaires	These are very routinely used in a variety of settings, particularly when working with other staff. Once set up they can be used repeatedly and results are collated automatically. They require very limited time from the facilitator and are cost-effective. They require an email address or some other means to send the link to participants. Not all participants will be used to working with electronic media. Response rates can be very low. Repeat or follow up surveys can be very useful to ascertain whether participants have managed to sustain behaviour change over a period of time (outcome evaluation). Knowing if other professionals have been able to implement changes into their working practice or not is extremely valuable information.
Quality-of-life measures	There are many validated tools designed to assess quality of life.	These measures consider the broad impact of behaviour change beyond clinical measures. They may look at the participants' emotional, psychological well-being, physical and social life and how that is affected. Such measures must have been tested for validity and reliability in order for the results to be meaningful. Consideration should always be given to whether the tool is appropriate for that specific participant group.

Table 7.4 (Continued)

Method	Examples	Considerations
		Some disease-specific quality of life scales are available.
		Some scales require the user to be registered prior to accessing information on how to score and analyse the tools.
		Some scales look at participants' abilities to undertake activities of daily living.
		Measures can assess functional ability, psychological well-being, social aspects, satisfaction with life or a combination of these.
		Quality-of-life measures are unlikely to be useful with one-off group education sessions but would be more appropriate with longer term programs.
		A comprehensive review of quality of life measurement scales is provided by Bowling (2005).
Food intake measures	These include food diaries and food frequency questionnaires, fruit and vegetable intake measures and bespoke measures related to specific aims.	Most of these measures will require a reasonable level of literacy and would need to be completed pre-and post any training session if they are to demonstrate change. Many participants tire easily of completing foods diaries and the level of accuracy in completion is extremely variable. Analysis of food diaries and food frequency questionnaires is time-consuming and requires specific skills and computer programmes. Focussing on one aspect of overall food intake may be appropriate, e.g. number of portions of fruit and vegetable consumed per day. All of these measures are likely to be self-reported and it must be considered that there are limitations and bias with this approach.
Physical activity questionnaires	There are many tools designed to measure physical activity and/ or sedentary behaviour and can be downloaded from the internet.	Need to consider the literacy level required. Some may require complex methods of analysis and are more suitable for research projects. Check if the tool is validated and is likely to give good quality data. Some sources of information include: – The Sedentary Behaviour Research Network provides information on a variety of tools that have been validated and could be used (www.sedentarybehaviour.org/sedentary-behaviour-questionnaires/, last accessed May 2016).

Table 7.4 (Continued)

Method	Examples	Considerations
		– The General Practice Physical Activity Questionnaire (GPPAQ) is a simple validated screening tool designed to assess the physical activity levels of adults and is available from www.gov.uk/government/ publications/general-practice-physical-activity-questionnaire-gppaq (last accessed May 2016). This indicates changes in the amount of time individuals spend on different activities such as specific exercise, active travel, walking, housework or gardening. – The Transport and Physical Activity Questionnaire (TPAQ) assesses the amount of time people spend in different domains activity and modes of transport (Adams *et al.,* 2014). This is not a comprehensive list.
Health literacy	There are a variety of measures available that can be used to measure health literacy.	The tool used must relate to the objectives of the session. Aspects that could be included might relate to the participants having knowledge about self-care, relevant medications, access to services, further information and support. If participants have difficulty with English language and literacy, then this may need to be done verbally rather than in a written format.
Other	Verbal feedback at the end of a session	Useful for getting an immediate response and for questions like 'what has been the most/ least helpful part of the session?' Participants may be reticent to talk in front of others.
	Post-its. Participants have Post-its to write key points on and stick them on a board as they leave.	Useful for brief feedback on questions like 'what went well?' and 'What could have been better?' Will not be able to measure all objectives or learning outcomes and may be quite superficial. Overcomes participant reticence for saying what they feel.

Challenges with evaluation

Although evaluation is clearly recognized as essential, it is important to acknowledge the limitations that can be faced in relation to group education and behaviour change. Lifestyle change is influenced by a multitude of factors and the full consequences of a change in lifestyle may take years to develop. Changes made may not be sustained for a variety of reasons. It is not possible to clearly link cause and long-term effect. It may be possible to demonstrate that an education session led to a change in knowledge or skill level and it may be possible to follow participants up for a few months and see changes in clinical outcomes but it is not likely to be possible to link this to long term lifestyle change that decreases health risk. There are too many other factors that affect behaviour. Similarly, with education of staff it is not likely that a facilitator will know that the education has impacted on how that staff member is interacting and advising patients, service users and carers in their day to day work. In some cases, linking with an academic partner can support the evaluation process and make it more rigorous and meaningful.

Ethical issues to consider

When working in healthcare there is always a need to consider what ethical issues are relevant to that scenario and evaluation of group education is no exception. Here are a few factors to consider:

- Be sensitive to the needs of the participants. Is what you are asking them to do appropriate and acceptable?
- Make sure you are preserving the anonymity of participants. In most cases evaluations will be anonymous and this is essential if participants are to feel able to express their views freely;
- Evaluate how worthwhile the education is. Resources must be used wisely and continuing to deliver material that is not effective is not ethical as it means that the resource is not available for more effective interventions;
- Consider the participant needs when choosing appropriate methods to collect data, for example literacy and language needs of the participants so that all have an opportunity to share their views;
- Report data collected and the analysis of that data faithfully;
- Draw appropriate conclusions from the data. It is good practice to discuss this with colleagues;
- Disseminating the findings of the evaluation, whether the education is well evaluated or not as this can inform future work.

Revising your session

If an evaluation is indicating that there are areas for improvement, then the session should be revised to try and address that. Sometimes a session will be delivered several times and then thoroughly reviewed based on the evaluation and sometimes the facilitator will revise it each time until there are consistently positive responses.

If a session is to be delivered frequently and by a number of facilitators, then it will cause confusion if different people keep changing minor details. There could end up being multiple copies of similar materials but not the consistency that is required. In this case a review date should be set for the materials to be revised and the collated evaluations to be reviewed. Even if evaluation is consistently positive any education session will need to be updated in relation to emerging evidence and new policy or guidance at least annually. Having resources marked clearly with a date of production and a date for review is good practice.

Presenting your results

Evaluations can be presented in a variety of formats and to a variety of audiences depending on the size of the education project, detail and format of the evaluation and the needs of stakeholders. Table 7.5 shows some possible formats and audiences for evaluation results.

Case Studies

Evaluation is an essential part of any education program whether it be a one-off session or series of sessions. There are many benefits to undertaking rigorous evaluation both for the facilitator and for participants, current and future. Evaluation needs to be tailored specifically to the intervention and the objectives that were set. This chapter has identified many of the issues to be considered.

Table 7.5 Formats for reporting evaluation results.

Possible audiences	Usual format of evaluation
Colleagues, both uni- and multi-professional meetings	Presentations, posters
Funders and other stakeholders, including patient groups	Short reports, presentations
Professional meetings and conferences	Abstracts, research papers and presentations, short reports

Case study 7.1 Healthy lifestyle group for people with learning disabilities

You have been asked to lead a project developing and delivering a series of eight group education sessions over a period of 4 months, including aspects of a healthy diet, physical activity, alcohol consumption and weight management. The target participants are an established group of 12 adults with learning disabilities who live supported in the community. The characteristics of the group are as follows:

- Age ranges from 22 to 54 years.
- Eight are female and four are male.
- Two are of South Asian ethnicity, one is African Caribbean and the others are white British.
- All are overweight or obese.
- None of the participants smoke.

As a group they are considered to be at increased cardiovascular risk.

The group meets twice a week (Tuesdays and Thursdays) from 10 am to 3 pm in a Community Centre and are supported by a community nurse and a support worker who specializes in working with people with learning disabilities.

The meals are planned and prepared by the group themselves and they choose what they are going to have a week in advance. They have rotas for shopping (with the support worker if needed), preparing the dining area, cooking, washing up and clearing the dining area. The community nurse and support worker are happy to work with you during the usual weekly contact time.

Questions

What other information would you need to help you plan this project?
What would be your overall aim and objectives for the project?
What would you do as:

1. Formative evaluation
2. Process evaluation
3. Short term impact evaluation
4. Longer term outcome evaluation?

What challenges would you anticipate with evaluation tools with this target group?

FACILITATOR APPROACH TO A HEALTHY LIFESTYLE GROUP FOR PEOPLE WITH LEARNING DISABILITIES

What other information would you need to help you plan this project?

It would be useful to obtain more background information on the participants such as:

- The level of literacy that is going to be appropriate for them as this will impact on the resources that can be used in the education sessions.
- The participants' social situations and in particular practical information such as who does the shopping and cooking in their households. It may be that they complete these activities themselves but some may have support and some may live with families or partners who undertake these roles.
- Income levels, which may be relatively low and therefore impact on the types of foods that are purchased.
- Where the participants live and the related access to shops and other food suppliers.
- Have they had any input around healthy lifestyle before?
- Do any of the participants have any other medical conditions that need to be considered such as diabetes or coeliac disease?
- Are there any religious and cultural issues that need to be considered which may impact on food intake or ability to undertake physical activity?
- Are there any other factors that may influence participants' ability to undertake physical activity?
- How many of them consume alcohol? It may be that some do not consume alcohol at all and that any information about alcohol only needs to be communicated to certain individuals.
- What would be your overall aim and objectives for the project?

The organization that funded the project is likely to have a specific agenda as to what they hope it will achieve. Other stakeholders such as the community nurse, support worker and indeed the participants themselves may have views that need to be considered. However, it is most likely to be that the overall aim will be to decrease participants' cardiovascular risk. The objectives should all contribute to that overall aim. They may therefore include supporting participants to:

- Increase physical activity levels (whenever that is possible with individual participants) to meet recommendations,
- Improve the nutritional balance of meals provided at the community centre,
- Make changes to dietary intake which are consistent with weight management and a cardioprotective diet,

- Avoid weight gain and ideally promote weight loss,
- Consume alcohol within recommended safe levels.

The learning outcomes for individual group education sessions should all be clearly related to these overall objectives and will need to incorporate specific changes in behaviour as well as knowledge related. For example, although it may be useful for participants to be able to describe the physical activity recommendations, it is of more importance that they increase their physical activity level. You may therefore want to set the learning outcome that says 'at the end of the education session (about physical activity) all participants who are physically able, will have a realistic and time specific and plan of how they are going to increase their physical activity level.

1. Formative evaluation

Formative evaluation would be very useful in this case. A clear understanding of the group participants' additional needs will support the facilitator to develop the project in line with those needs. For example, an understanding of the attention span of the participants will help the facilitator to plan how the sessions are going to be delivered and how long they can be. The participants may have very strong views about what works for them and what doesn't. Getting to know them and building a rapport with them will encourage them to share what is important to them. It is important to avoid making assumptions. A focus group is likely to be a positive way forward rather than using a method that requires more literacy skills. Working with the participants and their support workers, may also increase the likelihood of the changes being sustained after the intervention is completed. Participants may also be interested in particular subjects and it is important to build on their knowledge.

2. Process evaluation

As there are going to be eight individual sessions each of these will have specific learning outcomes and different teaching methods and resources. They will therefore need to be evaluated individually in relation to teaching methods that worked and those that need further development. As each session is undertaken the facilitator will need to monitor attendance and engagement and reflect on these prior to the following session. The participant aspect of this evaluation is likely to need to be verbal or use some other tools that require limited literacy. Stickers with smiley faces or frowning faces could be useful or participants could be asked to tick against activities that they like and put a cross on those they don't. Having a consistent approach to evaluation throughout the eight sessions may help participants to get used to the process. The community nurse and support worker may be able to support participants to complete this evaluation. It would also be important to capture the views of the community nurse and support worker as they know the participants better than the facilitator. They also may have many more ideas as to how behaviour change can be incorporated into their usual twice weekly meetings and what could be sustained over the long term.

3. Short-term impact evaluation

This will of course be related to the objectives of the project. There may be very many different ways of looking at this.

As the sessions have been delivered over a period of 4 months, it is possible that the group education has led to behaviour change and changes in clinical outcomes. Having the assistance of the community nurse and support worker may allow the facilitator to collect information pre-and post the group education such as body weight and BMI, waist circumference or blood pressure. This is extremely useful information which relates directly to the overall aim of the group education. Although these staff may be able to take blood to measure cholesterol levels or blood glucose these tests are costly, invasive and may cause distress to participants.

For many aspects of the impact evaluation it may be possible to use a variety of measures pre-and post the group education.

With physical activity it may be that participants would be very happy to use pedometers but may require assistance. It may be that their level of activity could be monitored pre-and post the group education using some kind of written format that takes into account the literacy needs of participants.

The facilitator could record information on the meals that are chosen and created by the group. This could give good insight into any changes that the group have accepted and tried to implement. For example, they may have chosen to limit or exclude high fat foods such as chips, pastry or creamy sauces. They may have increased the number of portions of fruits and vegetables that they provide or have decreased portions of less healthy options. Dietary analysis could be undertaken or simple qualitative aspects could be monitored.

Monitoring the overall food intake of the individuals could be very challenging due to the high level of literacy that is often required to either record or self-report food intake. Participants would most definitely require assistance with tools such as foods diaries or food frequency questionnaires and this may not be practical.

Knowledge could be measured using quizzes or questionnaires administered by the facilitator, community nurse or support worker.

4. Long-term outcome evaluation

As this group is established and likely to continue to meet on a regular basis it may well be possible to return and repeat measures that will assess how well the aim and objectives of the group education have been met in the long term. Such measures include body weight and BMI, physical activity levels, foods being prepared within the group and knowledge. It should always be acknowledged that other aspects external to the group education may have impacted on the behaviour change.

Case study 7.2 Nutrition training for school nurses

You have been given funding to deliver a series of nutrition updates for school nurses. These nurses locally have recently been given much more responsibility for weight management in the school environment. The format and content of the training has not been specified except that it needs to focus on prevention and management of childhood obesity.

What questions would you want to answer before embarking on the planning and delivery of this programme?

What challenges do you face in relation to the evaluation of this programme?

What type of impact would you wish to measure?

FACILITATOR APPROACH TO NUTRITION TRAINING FOR SCHOOL NURSES

What questions would you want to answer before embarking on the planning and delivery of this programme?

It would be really useful to undertake some needs assessment here and communicate with the nurses themselves and/or their managers. This could be done with focus groups, interviews with key staff or a survey. The following questions are examples of what could be helpful

What nutrition related issues do you encounter in your work? *There may be other issues that are related and need to be covered.*

What aspects of childhood obesity prevention and management would you like to learn more about? For example, National Child Measurement Programme, how to measure height and weight accurately in children, how to use BMI appropriately in children, speaking with parents about their child's weight, brief interventions, ways to increase physical activity levels, ideas for decreasing sedentary behaviours, ways to decrease energy intake, portion sizes for children, resources to support child weight management, local support groups, appropriate monitoring of children and so on.

As well as working out suitable content for the training session you might want to find out very practical details such as the best day of the week for training, best times of day (unless it is to be a whole day) and preferred locations.

What challenges do you face in relation to the evaluation of this programme?

With programmes like this it is usually relatively easy to evaluate process and impact as there will be no concerns over language and literacy and most people will be happy to complete an evaluation form on the day. In this case the facilitator will have to collate the responses manually, which can be time consuming and is often not completed due to time pressures. However, if the evaluation form is online you may get fewer people completing it and therefore a less complete response. The advantage of the online survey is that it will automatically collate the responses and there is no difficulty with reading the writing. Keep the evaluation focussed or people will not complete it. Mostly questions with tick box answers and some space for open text feedback is used. Most people do not want to write an essay at the end of the education session but they will also want enough space to write what is on their mind. This can be a frustration with online surveys where there is nowhere to explain what you mean or qualify your answer. Don't forget to pilot your evaluation survey to make sure that the questions make sense to other people!

What type of impact would you wish to measure?

The most important impact is whether the learning outcomes have been met and these could relate to knowledge, skills, confidence, awareness or attitude. For example, there could be learning outcomes relating to confidence and competency with measuring height and weight accurately, awareness of when to refer a child or family on to specialist services, knowledge of appropriate dietary and physical activity advice for the children and so on.

It will also be important to get the general feedback about the session, the venue, the teaching methods used, the facilitator skills, what was useful and what was less useful (if anything). It is always good if people have enjoyed the session but it also needs to be useful and giving new information.

References

Adams EJ, Goad M, Sahlqvist S, Bull FC, Cooper AR and Ogilvie D (2014). Reliability and Validity of the Transport and Physical Activity Questionnaire (TPAQ) for Assessing Physical Activity Behaviour. *PLoS ONE* 9(9): e107039. doi: 10.1371/journal.pone.0107039 (accessed 20 November 2015).

Bowling A (2005) *Measuring Health: A Review of Quality of Life Measurement Scales*, 3rd Edn. Maidenhead: Open University Press

Bowling A (2009). *Research Methods in Health: Investigating Health and Health Services*, 3rd Edn. Maidenhead: Open University Press.

Cavill N, Roberts K and Ells L (2015). *Evaluation of Weight Management, Physical Activity and Dietary Interventions: An Introductory Guide.* Oxford: Public Health England.

De Leeuw ED, Hox JJ and Dillman DA (2008). *International Handbook of Survey Methodology.* London: Lawrence Erlbaum Associates.

De Vaus D (2002). *Surveys in Social Research,* 5th Edn. London: Routledge.

Drummond MF, Sculpher MJ, Torrance GW, O'Brien BJ and Stoddart GL (2005). *Methods for the Economic Evaluation of Health Care Programmes.* Oxford: Oxford University Press.

Gillespie J, Midmore C, Hoeflich J, Ness C, Ballard P and Stewart L (2015). Parents as the start of the solution: a social marketing approach to understanding triggers and barriers to entering a childhood weight management service. *J Hum Nutr Diet* 28: 83–92.

Greaves C, Gillison F, Stathi A, *et al.* (2015) Waste the waist: a pilot randomised controlled trial of a primary care based intervention to support lifestyle change in people with high cardiovascular risk. *Int J Behav Nutr Phys Act* 12. Available at: DOI: 10.1186/s12966-014-0159-z.

Holli BB and Beto JA (2014). *Nutrition counseling and education skills for dietetics professionals,* 6th Edn. Baltimore: Lippincott, Williams and Wilkins.

McColl E, Jacoby A, Thomas L, *et al.* (2001). *Design and use of questionnaires: a review of best practice applicable to surveys of health service staff and patients. Health Technology Assessment* 5(31). Southampton: National Coordinating Centre for Health Technology Assessment.

Metzgar CJ, Preston AG, Miller DL and Nickols-Richardson SM (2014). Facilitators and barriers to weight loss and weight loss maintenance: a qualitative exploration. *J Hum Nutr Diet.* Available at: DOI: 10.1111/jhn.12273. [Accessed November 2015].

Naidoo J and Wills J (2009). *Foundations for Health Promotion,* 3rd Edn. London: Bailliere Tindall.

Newell R and Burnard P (2011). *Research for Evidence Based Practice in Healthcare,* 2nd Edn, Oxford: Wiley-Blackwell.

Rootman I, Goodstadt M and Hyndman B (eds) (2001). *Evaluation in Health Promotion: Principles and Perspectives.* Denmark: WHO.

Further reading

Cavill N, Roberts K and Ells L (2015). *Evaluation of Weight Management, Physical Activity and Dietary Interventions: An Introductory Guide.* Oxford: Public Health England.

Useful websites

NHS identity www.nhsidentity.nhs.uk/tools-and-resources/patient-information
The Information Standard, NHS England www.england.nhs.uk/tis/

Chapter 8 **Managing group interaction and how to overcome challenges**

Vanessa Halliday

8.1 Introduction

Previous chapters have focussed on how to plan and deliver education sessions that include activities to promote participant engagement. Using inclusive teaching techniques that take account of the learning styles and diverse characteristics of the group such as age, gender, culture, health conditions, intellectual ability and motivation is important. Using language and resources that are accessible to all participants will also help to engage the group. Whilst all of these things are essential for maintaining the participant's interest, how people interact and work together as a group will also influence how effective the session is at changing lifestyle behaviours for the better.

Within the context of this book, we are defining 'interaction' as what participants do when talking and engaging in conversation and discussion in order to share their knowledge, experiences and opinions with other members of the group. This chapter will focus on how you, as the facilitator, manage this group interaction. In particular, it will summarize ways to avoid and manage difficult circumstances and how to deal with participants that exhibit behaviours that you may find challenging. It will end with a discussion of how co-facilitators can work together to optimize group learning and interaction.

8.2 Facilitating group interaction

When a group of people meet for the first time, group interaction is not necessarily spontaneous. Most people find walking into a room of strangers daunting. Some will arrive just before the session is due to start to avoid having to make small talk whilst others will sit by themselves silently engrossed

How to Facilitate Lifestyle Change: Applying Group Education in Healthcare, First Edition.
Amanda Avery, Kirsten Whitehead and Vanessa Halliday.
© 2017 John Wiley & Sons, Ltd. Published 2017 by John Wiley & Sons, Ltd.

in their mobile phone. There are of course others that relish the opportunity to talk about their life and health conditions and who will immediately interact with anyone that is in the room. The point is that, as a facilitator, don't assume that the people attending your session will want to talk to each other or even be expecting that they have to. It is your job to facilitate interaction and, in some cases, this can be hard work.

As previously highlighted, greeting participants warmly is the first step in helping to create a positive learning environment where people feel confident and able to contribute. Icebreaker activities will also help the group get to know each other and set the tone for the level of interaction that will be required from them. It is likely that what follows will be a combination of the facilitator communicating information to the group, proposing new ideas and stimulating or moderating discussion. The primary aim of these activities is to empower the group and individual participants to be able to reflect on their own experiences and behaviours, with a view to identifying ways that they can make positive lifestyle changes. In addition to what has previously been discussed in Chapter 3 with regards to the importance of using effective communication skills and emotional intelligence when facilitating sessions, Box 8.1 provides a summary of how to manage group interaction.

Box 8.1 Managing group interaction

Establishing group interaction

In order to manage group interaction, you first need to create an environment where people feel able to speak and contribute. Greet participants warmly and learn their preferred names (or use name badges). Think about how your own body language and facial expressions are being perceived by the group. First impressions are important in establishing a positive rapport.

Maintaining group interaction

Once you have people talking you need to make sure that they continue to contribute and grow in confidence. This in itself may be enough to draw others into the conversation. Use discussion generating questions 'What is your experience of...?', 'What is your opinion on...?' and probing questions: 'What exactly do you mean by that?' 'Can you explain in more detail about...?', to stimulate further discussion. Make sure you are maintaining eye contact with different members of the group and consciously look around for other people that look like they might want to contribute. Encourage and respect all views and contributions.

> **Monitoring group interaction**
>
> Taking time to monitor how participants are interacting with the session, and with each other, is important. Particularly when you are new to this type of facilitation role, it can be a challenge to do this when you are presenting. Make a conscious effort to look around the group at regular intervals. What do people's body language or facial expressions tell you? Are they smiling and nodding which suggests they are content and in agreement with what is being discussed or are they staring out of the window, shaking their head or frowning? If most of the group look disengaged think about what could be the reasons for this. If in doubt, acknowledge the fact that people are looking confused or distracted and ask why. It might be that an important point has been misunderstood or simply that it is time for a refreshment break. Depending on the length of the session asking for mid-programme feedback from the group can be a good way of gauging how things are going.

8.3 Cultural sensitivity in group education

It is likely that for many of you, the participants attending your group will be culturally diverse. This might be in terms of their ethnicity, religion or socio-economic status but also other characteristics such as age, gender, health status and sexual orientation. Cultural competence can be defined as 'a set of congruent behaviours, attitudes and policies that come together in a system, agency, or amongst professionals and enables that system, agency, or those professionals to work effectively in cross-cultural situations' (Cross *et al.*, 1989). Unsurprisingly, research suggests that the cultural competence of health care professionals can positively influence health related outcomes (Horvat *et al.*, 2014). In addition to this, creating a comfortable environment where all participants feel able to learn, means that cultural awareness and cultural sensitivity is important for you to consider when delivering your sessions.

> **TOP TIPS FOR DEMONSTRATING CULTURAL COMPETENCE AND SENSITIVITY**
>
> - Take time to reflect and understand your own cultural beliefs, attitudes and values.
> - Avoid making assumptions and stereotyping; be non-judgemental and respectful.
> - Demonstrate that you are interested in hearing and learning about others' culture by actively listening.

- Check that what you are saying is being understood.
- Where required, work with interpreters or if possible, bilingual staff.
- Use the first-person tense, for example 'person with diabetes' rather than 'diabetic person' and avoid using labels, for example 'diabetics'.
- Consider your level of formality and if any of your questions could be culturally insensitive or inappropriate.
- If you are providing food make sure that it is culturally appropriate.
- Plan your timetable and venue so that it takes into account, for example, of religious prayer times.
- Work with local community workers in local community venues to help establish familiarity and rapport within the group.

Further reading, including a cultural competence self-assessment checklist (Sutton, 2000).

8.4 How to manage discussion of sensitive subjects

There are likely to be times when the subject being discussed unavoidably involves talking about sensitive material. This may be in terms of a planned topic or activity or it could be identified and brought into the conversation by one of the group members. How you manage these situations requires careful consideration if you are to avoid inadvertently upsetting members of the group. There is not a definitive list of examples of what could be potentially distressing material as it will be dependent on the individuals that you have in the group. Whereas there are more obvious topics such as death, drug and alcohol abuse, relationships and mental health that some groups may find sensitive, other subjects, such as cancer, could be upsetting to an individual that has recently been bereaved.

If you are aware that what you will be discussing could potentially be upsetting then highlighting this at the start of the session, and again just before you introduce the topic, can be helpful. Including something in the ground rules or agreement for working together, around personal experiences and disclosure may also be relevant. Giving participants the choice of stepping out of the room is one option, although you should be aware that some will feel that this in itself is distressing. If sensitive issues arise unexpectedly acknowledging that what is being discussed could be upsetting or controversial and giving the group the opportunity to express their thoughts, is important. Should you be aware of a member of the group becoming upset you may choose to halt the discussion and, if appropriate, suggest taking a short break. If members of the group do have to leave the session, following this up with them to ask how they are, is important. Having a list of organizations that you can signpost people to for additional support can also be useful.

8.5 Avoiding challenging situations

As previously established in this book, learning as a group provides many opportunities and benefits for participants. Education sessions can be a forum where participants are able to voice and share their own experiences as well as hearing from others in similar situations. These discussions can provide them with a strong sense of 'not being the only one', which may in turn help them to put their problems into perspective. Hearing how others have managed their condition, dealt with problems and made positive changes can also be useful. However, there may be some situations where group members disagree with what is being said and, although mild confrontation can help individuals develop their own thoughts and understanding, conflict within the room can be detrimental to the education process.

8.6 Working with group members that exhibit behaviours that you find challenging to manage

Most of the time you will be involved in educating individuals who are polite, respectful and motivated to participate. However, from time to time there will be a small number of 'challenging' group members. When this happens, as the group facilitator, you should be prepared with strategies in place to handle these situations. Good ground rules, which have been agreed from the onset by all group members, are particularly important in these situations and should be referred to. Ground rules should be viewed as a contract and you may choose to ask members to sign a copy once the group is formed. If a member is unable to stick to these rules, then they can be asked to leave the group if their behaviour is jeopardizing the productive environment.

Occasionally conflict may occur when participants have strong and opposing ideas on a subject. A facilitator needs to be sensitive to possible differences and tensions in the group and encourage people to work through these, reminding people of their common goals. If the conflict is not related to the programme, then it is important to ask members to put the issue to one side and to discuss outside the group setting.

Dominant members can also be disruptive to the functioning of a group. Sometimes there is one person who dominates the discussions, confident that they have all the right answers. A good facilitator needs to make sure that everyone has equal opportunities to speak and are not overshadowed. An important ground rule is to make this clear from the formation of the group. Strategies can be to give that person additional responsibility, to split the group into smaller groups and place similar types of people together or to ask people to take turns to make comments.

In contrast, there will be group members who are quite shy or afraid to express their opinions in a group. The most effective way of encouraging people who are shy is to empower them by referring back and using their ideas so they know they are important and valued. Alternatively, they may also be given additional responsibility such as note-taking and summarizing feedback. It is always worth trying to establish a reason for silence.

Table 8.1 describes the characteristics and behaviours that group members may exhibit that can be challenging for the facilitator to manage. It also gives examples of how the facilitator may approach these situations.

Table 8.1 How to manage participants that exhibit behaviours that can be challenging.

Characteristic	Challenging behaviour	Facilitator approach
Dominant monopoliser or eager beaver	Contributes at every opportunity. May be very keen to answer every question or just likes the sound of their own voice	• After they have made their first point thank them for their contribution and ask if anyone else has something to say. • Focus on encouraging participation from all members of the group by directing questions to, e.g., specific people or areas of the room. • Split the main group into smaller groups for specific tasks.
Expert	Believes that they already know it all	• If they appear to be genuinely knowledgeable, establish what their background is and use their contributions positively. • If their expertise is self-perceived, recognize the factual points but tactfully challenge speculation or theory.
Side-tracker	Has their own agenda and diverts the discussion to it at every occasion	• Be direct by acknowledging that their point is interesting but making it clear that due to time pressure there is a need to focus on the main issue. • If relevant, offer to speak to them about the issue at the break or the end of the session. • Be aware that in many cases, if this type of participants does not feel like their point has been heard, they will continue to voice it.
Clown	Constantly makes a joke of what is being said	• If possible, acknowledge and summarize any serious points that their joke contributes. • If you cannot see any relevance ask them to clarify this 'On a serious note, could you clarify the point that you are making please?'

(Continued)

Table 8.1 (Continued)

Characteristic	Challenging behaviour	Facilitator approach
Heckler	Interrupts with unhelpful and possibly rude or embarrassing comments	• Ask them if they have a question that they would like to ask. • Where necessary acknowledge that their comments are unhelpful or offensive. • In some situations, it may be necessary to inform them that if they continue with their unhelpful comments they will be asked to leave the group. You may choose to do this discretely at one of the breaks.
Argumentative	Appears hostile and contradicts what you and others are saying at every opportunity	• Stay calm and avoid getting drawn into an argument. • If possible, rephrase what they have said in a more objective way. • Avoid lengthy debate: 'Can we agree to disagree on this point?' • Ask for other participants' opinions in an attempt to establish a balanced view of the 'argument'. • If the debate is between two members of the group draw other participants into the discussion 'What do other people think about this?' • In extreme situations where a participant is being aggressive it may be necessary to warn them that if they continue with that behaviour they will be asked to leave the group. Following this, if the situation does not improve, you will need to remove them from the group.
Complainer	Persistently negative about what is being discussed or about a previous experience	• Ask them to be specific about what their point or complaint is. • Acknowledge the relevance and legitimacy where appropriate. • Enthusiastically giving them encouragement and credit for their contribution can help to prevent ongoing negativity. • Ask other members of the group for their opinion or experience. • Avoid getting side-tracked.
Silent	Does not contribute	• Encourage them to contribute by making eye contact. • Speaking to them at break times may help you identify the reason behind why they are quiet. • Statements such as 'I'm interested in hearing the thoughts from those people that haven't spoken yet' may help draw them into the conversation.

(Continued)

Table 8.1 (Continued)

Characteristic	Challenging behaviour	Facilitator approach
Shy or timid	Attempts to contribute but is quietly spoken and lacks confidence	• Encourage their contribution by using minimal encouragers such as nodding your head and saying 'yes, go on...'. • Direct simpler questions towards them. • Challenge other members of the group that try to interrupt 'It is an important point that John is making, please let him finish what he is saying'. • Ask the group to discuss questions by working in pairs.
Reticent	May have the confidence to participate but appears disengaged or withdrawn	• It can be helpful to reflect on if they entered the session with a reticent attitude or if it developed as a consequence of something that was said. • Asking them to contribute by sharing their opinion or experience may help to re-engage them. • What is important to them about this subject? • Speaking to them at break times may help you identify the reason behind their behaviour.
Disruptive	Talks or whispers to those sat next to them	• Stop the session and try to make eye contact with them. • If they do not take this hint, politely ask them if there is something that they don't understand or to share their thoughts with the rest of the group.

8.7 Answering questions and maintaining your credibility when challenged

Establishing your credibility as an educator is important. It is likely that taking the time at the start of the session to highlight your experience and why you are there, along with acting professionally and being well organized, will prevent any serious challenges of your credibility. Particularly if you are new to this type of facilitation role, it is helpful for you to understand that participants will ask questions, some of which you will be able to answer with confidence and others that you won't. There are also likely to be many situations where there will not necessarily be one definitive response. All of these scenarios are completely normal.

Aside from the healthy questioning from participants, in some situations you may feel that your credibility is being questioned if a member of the group persistently challenges the point that you are making or, on the very

---

TOP TIPS FOR HOW TO RESPOND TO QUESTIONS THAT YOU DON'T KNOW THE ANSWER TO

It goes without saying that if you are not confident about the answer to a question don't guess or make it up as this is the quickest way to lose credibility. Instead be honest 'That's a really [good/important/interesting] question. I am not sure that I know the answer'. You can then either ask the person who posed the question what their thoughts are or open it up to the group. If at the end of the discussion the question remains unanswered you can let the group know that you will look into it further following the session. Bear in mind that depending on if this is a one off session, you will need to have some method of contacting participants after the event to inform them of the answer. Alternatively, you may have the time during the session to do some research on the internet or 'phone a friend'!

---

rare occasion, blatantly tells you that you are wrong. If this happens it is important to keep calm and not get defensive. It is good practice to reflect on whether the information that you are sharing is accurate. Is it based on scientific research, your experience or your opinion? Being clear to participants about which one of these it is, is important. Likewise, if it is a controversial subject area then highlight this to the group and give them the chance to express their views. As discussed previously, asking other participants for their opinions and experience can also help resolve the situation. Ultimately, it may be necessary in some situations to 'agree to disagree' with the individual who is challenging the point.

Challenging participants' misconceptions

Given the abundance of information in the news and on the internet, it is not surprising that the general public are often confused about what constitutes a healthy diet and lifestyle. As a consequence, participants in your groups are likely to share with you their, sometimes, mis-informed beliefs. It is important for the individual, and the rest to the group, that these misconceptions do not go unchallenged, otherwise you run the risk of perpetuating the 'myth'. Case Study 8.1 next, gives an example of how a facilitator could manage this type of situation.

Case study 8.1 Challenging participants' misconceptions

You are facilitating a weight management group education session that is being held in a community health centre located in an area of high unemployment and deprivation. During the session one of the participants, Julia, tells you that she has been eating a grapefruit every day for the last 6 years as it helps to 'burn fat'. As the facilitator, how would you manage this scenario?

FACILITATOR APPROACH TO CHALLENGING PARTICIPANTS' MISCONCEPTIONS

It is important to first acknowledge the point that Julia has made and thank her for sharing the information with the group. Given the lack of scientific evidence confirming how grapefruit 'burns fat' in humans, it is important to explore how she came to believe this to be the case. This needs to be done sensitively as it is something that she has been doing for many years and so is likely to have strong feelings about. Finding out where Julia got the information from originally can be helpful when formulating your response. Giving a balanced argument as to why people choose to include grapefruit in their diets could be helpful. For example, the advantages of the fibre and vitamin C content and enjoyment of eating the fruit versus the cost and potential for some drug interactions, particularly if taken as grapefruit juice. You do, however, need to be clear to Julia, and the rest of the group, that grapefruit is not recommended to aid weight loss in this way.

8.8 Managing the use of mobile devices

In today's society most people have a mobile telephone and some may also have an IPad or tablet device that they carry around with them. As identified in Chapter 5, a discussion on the expectations about the use of mobile devices should be included along with other ground rules at the start of the session. For example, a reasonable agreement might be that all mobile devices are switched to silent with only urgent calls being answered outside of the room. This does not, however, account for people who are distracted from the session by emails or social media. Whilst you may request that participants wait until the breaks to read and respond to their emails, in some cases using mobile devices during the session to make notes or use the internet to clarify points that are being made, can enhance learning. This is something that needs to be balanced alongside the potential for distracting the facilitator and possibly other participants.

Although most of the time group members will respect the ground rules, there may be some situations where participants continue to use their mobile devices for reasons that are outside the purpose of the session. Those of you that are experienced facilitators may be familiar with participants having one, or in some cases two, mobile phones on the table next to them, answering emails and in extreme situations holding telephone calls during sessions. When this happens it is important to challenge the behaviour quickly. This can be done by stopping the session and making eye contact with them. Usually this will be enough for them to realize that their behaviour is distracting. If not it may be necessary to politely ask them if what they are doing is urgent, to take the call outside or to wait until the break or after the session.

8.9 Timekeeping

Keeping the session running to time is important for a number of reasons. Having to rush through material can lead to an unsatisfactory experience for all concerned whilst running over time may mean that you do not cover all of the learning outcomes. There are also practical reasons why the session must end on time. The room could be booked by someone else, the facilitator may have a later engagement or the participants may have childcare or transport arranged.

Developing a lesson plan that is appropriate for the length of the session is clearly an important element of time management, as is ensuring group activities don't overrun. Whilst both of these things are relatively straightforward for the facilitator to control, managing participants timekeeping can be more of a challenge.

Making sure that pre-session participant information includes start and finish times, along with the expectation that people are expected to attend the full session, is important. However, there will always be some unavoidable circumstances that lead to participants arriving late to the session or having to leave early and facilitators should be sympathetic to these events. If there are a number of people missing at the time the session is scheduled to start you may choose to wait for a few minutes. Delaying the start any more than this can be frustrating for those that did arrive on time and can also have a knock on effect with regards to finishing. What does need to be addressed is when participants are persistently late in getting to the session or returning after refreshment breaks. As discussed previously, including timekeeping in the discussion of ground rules can help to avoid this situation. It is, however, possible that persistent offenders missed this discussion due to their tardiness! Politely reminding the group of the importance of arriving promptly is usually enough to avoid the situation being repeated. Where this is not the case, speaking to the offending members of the group individually can help. In extreme circumstances to avoid disruptions you may decide that individuals who arrive more than, for example, 10 minutes late will not be admitted.

8.10 Getting people to attend

So far we have focussed on how to manage difficult situations during the education session. You may, however, experience problems before it begins, as in some circumstances getting people to attend can be a challenge. There are numerous reasons why people may choose not to attend your session. At structured group education sessions for those recently diagnosed with type 2 diabetes, shame and stigma around the diagnosis, practical inconvenience of the session and lack of perceived benefit have been highlighted as important in the decision-making process (Winkley *et al.*, 2015a). It is also possible that the people who are most likely to benefit from your session, such as those who smoke and have poorer glycaemic control, are the ones that need the most encouragement to attend (Winkley *et al.*, 2015b).

The section on recruitment of participants in Chapter 4 of this book identifies ways that you can make sure that you optimize the targeting and advertising of your education sessions. If you are aware that you need to recruit more hard to reach groups, or those that are more likely to be reluctant to attend, take additional time to consider how best to use a combination of approaches. This could include traditional routes such as posters, flyers and referrals from staff that work with potential participants. You may also wish to consider posting the information online on local websites and web-based forums as well as using social media, such as Facebook and Twitter, to advertise the event.

Over recent years there has been increasing interest in how incentives can be used to encourage health related behaviour change, with positive incentives proving more effective than when penalties are imposed (Lynagh *et al.*, 2013). Dependent on your own local guidelines and policies, budget available and personal views, this may be something that you wish to consider. Whether or not you decide to offer a financial incentive or vouchers, entry into a 'prize draw' or simply the meal to take home after the cook and eat session, making sure that you are clear to potential participants what is the personal benefit to them, could help boost your attendance rates.

8.11 Group dynamics

As highlighted earlier, it is likely that you will be educating groups that are made up of participants from diverse backgrounds whether that be age, culture, social or educational experiences. For this reason, it is inevitable that they will have different opinions and ideas. Those of you who are experienced facilitators will be able to remember times when you have delivered the same education session, in the same way but to different groups. You may have walked away with completely different perceptions on how the session went. It is likely that group dynamics were playing a part in what happened and understanding how this happened is an important role for the facilitator.

In Chapter 3, the Tuckman model of group development (Tuckman, 1965) was discussed. Awareness of this model (forming, storming, norming, performing), in the context of group dynamics, can be helpful when trying to understand and manage group interaction. Particularly when you are facilitating a series of sessions over a longer period of time, you may be able to attribute any problems or conflicts within the group to the stage of development. Acknowledgement of this can be helpful in deciding if it is a 'normal' part of the process that will pass or something more serious that needs addressing. However, if you are only involved with a group for a one-off short session, group development processes may be less relevant. Nonetheless, you should still be able to identify the positive or negative dynamic within the group.

Examples of positive group dynamic behaviour:
- Group members are happy to interact and share their experiences and ideas
- Participants trust and respect one another
- Participation in group activities is enthusiastic and productive.

Examples of negative group dynamic behaviour:
- There is limited interaction between participants
- Discussion is negative and complaining
- Group members engage in discussion and activities reluctantly and are unproductive
- Members of the group are disruptive.

Influencing group dynamics

Research suggests that groups have the potential to influence individuals' actions, thoughts and feelings (Forsyth, 2010). As a facilitator you are also a member of the group that you are working with and, as such you play a part in the dynamic. The process of this is likely to be different in each situation due to the inherent personality traits of the individuals and the unique situation that arises when they are forced to interact as a group. However, there are actions that the facilitator can take in an attempt to make sure that the dynamic of the group does not disrupt the learning environment. First and foremost, the attitude and behaviour of the facilitator can set the tone. Imagine an enthusiastic and confident facilitator that exudes energy compared to one that is timid, disorganized or apologetic. It is more likely that a facilitator with the latter characteristics will contribute to a negative group dynamic. Secondly, consciously observing the group for examples of inappropriate behaviour and tackling the issue quickly can stop the problem escalating. Members of the group with dominant characteristics, such as those that are monopolizing the conversation, being argumentative or disruptive, can heavily influence the group dynamic so it is important to address this sooner rather than later. Finally, when using breakout groups, identifying who works well together and who doesn't. Splitting the larger group up accordingly may help foster positivity.

8.12 Working with co-facilitators

Depending on the type of activities included in the session, or size of the group, it may be appropriate for there to be more than one facilitator. Having two or more facilitators has many advantages such as sharing the preparation workload and having a wider breadth of knowledge and expertise. Facilitating an education session can be physically and mentally tiring so having more than one person contributing to the session can help to keep up the energy levels and enthusiasm of the group. It will also mean that for participants the presentation voice and style will be varied. Practically, an additional facilitator can help with preparing the room, welcoming participants, giving out resources and supervising small group activities. The non-presenting facilitator may also be in a better position to gauge the reaction and mood of the participants during sessions.

What to consider when working with co-facilitators

In contrast to the advantages that co-facilitation can bring there are challenges that can arise when working with others. Consideration of the following points should help to avoid any co-facilitator conflicts.

Before the session
If it is a new session that is being developed, try to involve all facilitators in the planning and preparation stages. This way you will be able to share the tasks equally and make sure that you are playing to everyone's strengths when it comes to agreeing who will deliver each activity. Agree the aim and objectives of the session along with when you will meet to discuss progress.

It is helpful if notes are made as an aide memoire during each meeting and circulated with required actions highlighted.

Where possible work with people that you know will complement your own presentation style. Observing other facilitators in action can be a good way to do this. Alternatively, where this is not possible, have an open conversation where you discuss your own approach, experiences, strengths and limitations, along with the types of activities that you enjoy facilitating. If you are aware of differing opinions between co-facilitators related to the subject material discuss how you will manage them. This will avoid confusing participants with inconsistencies during the session. It will also avoid public disagreements.

When preparing for the session be clear about who is responsible for each task, for example, who will prepare and bring the resources or organize the refreshments? Rather than just communicating this verbally, make sure it is documented and circulated to avoid things being missed. Importantly, agree how you will facilitate the session. For example, are you happy for co-facilitators to interrupt and add any points you have missed, voice their opinions or ask questions to you or participants? How will you let each other know if activities are running over time? Overall, you need to be clear on the lesson plan regarding who will lead each section and activity. It can look unprofessional if it appears that facilitators are unsure, or if the decision has to be made on the spot.

During the session

Ongoing and open communication between facilitators can help the session run smoothly. Take opportunities during breaks and group activities to catch up with each other on how the session is running. Giving positive feedback and reassurance at these points will result in a supportive environment for those presenting and can improve the experience for all involved.

During the activities that you are observing, if there is additional information that you want to add, do it in a way that supports your co-facilitator 'That is a really important point that Sarah has made, I also have experience of where that has worked...'. Likewise, if you are aware of something that has been missed, or that participants are looking confused following an explanation, acknowledge this. For example, 'I just wanted to expand on what Sarah said about...'. When facilitating an activity, you can also involve your co-facilitator by asking if they have anything further to add.

After the session

Plan time for a post-session debrief. Ideally, a short discussion straight after to capture any immediate reflections can be helpful. This should then be followed up with a meeting at a later date where the participant evaluations are scrutinized and any necessary changes to the session are suggested and discussed. Be honest about what you felt went well and what could be improved including in your discussion reflections on both the content and facilitation approach. This can help not only improve the session, but also your and your co-facilitator skills.

References

Cross TL, Bazron BJ, Dennis KW and Isaacs MR (1989). *Towards a Culturally Competent System of Care* [Online]. Available from: http://files.eric.ed.gov/fulltext/ED330171.pdf [Accessed May 2016].

Forsyth DR (2010). *Group Dynamics*, 5th Edn. Belmont, CA: Wadsworth Cengage Learning.

Horvat L, Horey D, Romios P and Kis-Rigo J (2014). Cultural competence education for health professionals. *Cochrane Database of Systematic Reviews* 5: CD009405. Available from: DOI: 10.1002/14651858.CD009405.pub2. [Accessed November 2015].

Lynagh MC, Sanson-Fisher RW and Bonevski B (2013). What's Good for the Goose is Good for the Gander. Guiding principles for the use of financial incentives in health behaviour change. *Int J Behav Med* 20: 114–120.

Tuckman BW (1965). Developmental sequence in small groups. *Psychol Bull* 63(6): 384–399.

Winkley K, Evwierhoma C, Amiel SA, Lempp HK, Ismail K and Forbes A (2015a). Patient explanations for non-attendance at structured diabetes education sessions for newly diagnosed type 2 diabetes: A qualitative study. *Diabetic Med* 32(1): 120–128.

Winkley K, Stahl D, Chamley M, Stopford R, Boughdady M *et al.* (2015b). Low attendance at structured education for people with newly diagnosed type 2 diabetes: General practice characteristics and individual patient factors predict uptake. *Patient Educ Couns*. Available from: www.sciencedirect.com/science/article/pii/S0738399115300525 [Accessed September 2015].

Further reading

Jacques D and Salmon G (2007). *Learning in Groups: A Handbook for Face-to-Face and Online Environments*. London: Routledge.

Forsyth DR (2010). *Group Dynamics*, 5th Edn. Belmont CA: Wadsworth Cengage Learning.

Sutton M (2000). Improving patient care cultural competence. *Fam Pract Manag* 7(9): 58–60. Available from: www.aafp.org/fpm/2000/1000/p58.html [Accessed May 2016].

Chapter 9 **Personal development in group facilitation skills**

Amanda Avery

9.1 Introduction

It has already been suggested that it is very important to feel comfortable about one's knowledge of the subject material and the supporting current evidence base. This cannot be over-emphasized and it can also be helpful to be aware of how recent scientific findings have been portrayed by the media – what messages have the public received on certain topics? Some of the messages portrayed by the media may have been quite confusing. For example, should we have more fat and less carbohydrate in our diet? Are e-cigarettes really a better substitute? Is some alcohol good and protective against heart disease or are some types of exercise more valuable for us than others? The group facilitator needs to be aware of all of these debates. Therefore, continuing professional development in specific subject areas is going to enhance the group participants' confidence in the competencies of the group facilitator.

Some facilitators will be fortunate to have personal traits that mean that they find it relatively easy to facilitate an effective group session – or at least it may seem that this is the case to the observer. For example, they may naturally be a 'people person' who easily interacts with new people making them feel welcomed and included. Other people may have to work at developing their group facilitation skills.

Irrespective of current level of skills and confidence, continuing personal development in the area of facilitating group education is really important. The rest of this chapter will focus on the different methods that can be used.

How to Facilitate Lifestyle Change: Applying Group Education in Healthcare, First Edition.
Amanda Avery, Kirsten Whitehead and Vanessa Halliday.
© 2017 John Wiley & Sons, Ltd. Published 2017 by John Wiley & Sons, Ltd.

9.2 Reflection

Reflective practice is widely regarded as an essential ingredient in professional development. We can learn and improve through experience. Reflection is a form of self-evaluation (Askew, 2004). It is always useful to reflect on how a group session went as soon as possible after the facilitation. Again some people are natural reflectors whilst others are not. Yet this is one of the most accessible methods to support personal development. In its simplified form reflection is all about 'What', 'So What' and 'What Next' (Driscoll, 2007). So after a group session the facilitator should be thinking about what happened, what they felt went particularly well and what they felt could have gone better and as a consequence what they will do differently next time. There may have been some particular circumstances that affected why things went as they did and the reflection process should capture what they would do differently if these same circumstances should arise. It is also useful to capture the evaluation of the session in the reflection process allowing time to really study the responses and think about the context in which the responses have been made and feed this into the 'So What'.

A reflection template could be used and people who are new to facilitating group sessions may find this particularly helpful to complete and have in their professional development portfolio. The headings and subheadings used by Gibbs (1988) in their Reflective Cycle could be useful to use in the template (Figure 9.1). These headings give a little more depth to the 'What', So What' and 'What Next' and lead into an Action Plan.

If co-facilitating a group programme, it is good practice to schedule a co-facilitator de-brief and to jointly reflect on what happened, what went well and what you might do differently next time, taking into consideration the evaluations also and again to document any actions that it is felt are required.

The action plan may include the perceived need for additional training in a particular area, as discussed later in this chapter, or other forms of professional development such as making time available to research a certain topic.

The evaluative responses from the group members have been included as an important part of the reflection process. It may be helpful to ask an independent person to analyse the evaluation forms as they are likely to be more objective about the responses.

9.3 Peer observation

A very easy way to improve delivery style and content is to seek **peer observation**. Peer observation can be undertaken by a colleague who is from the same background but this does not need to be the case – it could be someone from a completely different background and this can have some advantages. For example, the peer observer could be both a healthcare professional skilled in

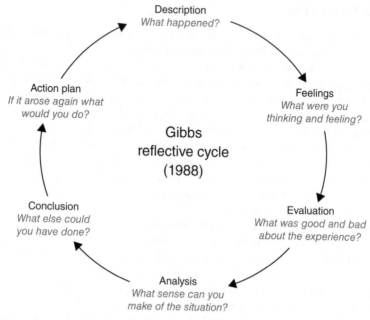

Figure 9.1 Gibbs Reflective Cycle, source Gibbs (1988).

group facilitation but who is not familiar with the particular lifestyle behaviour and so is taking on board the information as a member of the group would be. Alternatively, it could be that a mentor is asked to provide feedback.

Having standardized peer observation feedback forms can be helpful to both the person being observed and the observer (examples are provided in Boxes 9.1, 9.2 and 9.3). Box 9.1 is an example of a form which could be completed by the group facilitator who is being observed and given in advance to the peer observer. It is useful for the person observing the session to have some information in advance about the session to be observed. This information could include the aim and objectives of the session, the desired learning outcomes for the participants and any specific areas that the facilitator would like feedback on. Following the observation, it is helpful to receive both verbal and written feedback. Box 9.2 is an example of a form that could be completed by the observer either during or immediately after the session and is used as part of the verbal feedback with the person being observed. The written feedback, alongside some reflections (Box 9.3), can be kept in one's personal development portfolio and used as a developmental tool.

If peer review, observation and mentoring are undertaken on a regular basis and in a supportive environment, then they become much more comfortable and less of a threat. Some healthcare professionals do find peer

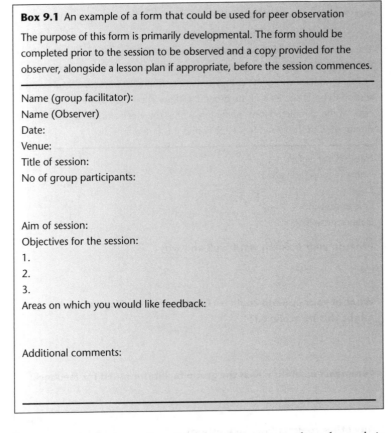

Box 9.1 An example of a form that could be used for peer observation

The purpose of this form is primarily developmental. The form should be completed prior to the session to be observed and a copy provided for the observer, alongside a lesson plan if appropriate, before the session commences.

Name (group facilitator):

Name (Observer)

Date:

Venue:

Title of session:

No of group participants:

Aim of session:

Objectives for the session:

1.

2.

3.

Areas on which you would like feedback:

Additional comments:

observation threatening and can become quite anxious perhaps due to their own lack of self-efficacy. The ideal situation is for the group facilitator also to have the opportunity to be an observer and to be able to provide constructive feedback to someone else. Observing or shadowing is a great way to improve one's own facilitation style and can complement reflective practice. Observers benefit from the exposure to someone else's practice and philosophy, with the opportunity to reflect on their own (Blackwell, 1996).

Collegiate Observation, Enquiry and Discussion (COED)

COED provides a framework that enables those who are involved in any teaching activity, including facilitating group education, to develop individual and collegiate practice in learning and teaching. Colleagues are uniquely placed to provide constructive and useful feedback on all aspects of teaching and learning from planning and organizing, to methods of delivery and evaluation (Blackwell, 1996). De Stobbeleir *et al.* (2011) found that staff who

Box 9.2 An example of a form that could be used for peer observation (Observer's feedback form)

The purpose of this form is primarily developmental. Please read the preparation form before observing the session and completing this form.

This form itself should be completed either during or immediately after the session to be observed and the group facilitator should be provided with a copy of the completed form preferably within the week and the session discussed with the group facilitator within this time frame also.

Name (Observer):
Name (Group facilitator):
Date:
Title of session:
Date of session:

What in your opinion went well and why?

What in your opinion could be improved or developed? How might this be achieved?

Comments on areas which the group facilitator asked for feedback:

Any other comments or suggestions:

sought direct feedback or feedback from a variety of sources exhibited more creativity in their work.

In order to provide a high quality learning experience for group participants it is essential that facilitators engage in ongoing professional development in learning and teaching, sharing practice with one another, perhaps at team 'away days'. This may include:

- reporting on an example of good practice and nominating facilitators for healthcare awards
- areas for development can be identified and provision made for appropriate support and development

Box 9.3 An example of a form that could be used by the group facilitator to reflect on both the written and verbal comments received from the observer (A copy to be kept in personal portfolio, alongside forms from Boxes 9.1 and 9.2 and a copy to be sent back to the observer).

What were the most important points to emerge from the feedback received from the observer?

What changes will you make as a result of the feedback (to both the particular session and to other sessions if applicable)?

Reflective comments about the observation.

- dedicated forums for staff to come together and talk about and develop their group facilitation skills.

What does COED involve?

Teams are expected to ensure that all members involved in facilitating group education engage in some form of activity with peers that facilitates the development of learning and teaching practice. This could be through some form of peer observation and feedback, through enquiry into individual practice, to playing an active role in departmental discussions about different

TOP TIP: COLLEGIATE DISCUSSION

- Simple straightforward conversations with colleagues are a valuable, often overlooked source of professional development in all aspects of teaching and learning. They offer a valuable opportunity to discuss and share different ideas and practices.
- Some interesting things can come from talking with colleagues and seeing things from their point of view.
- Regular, supportive feedback and discussions can help people new to facilitating integrate better into their new role (Morrison, 1993).

methods, styles and approaches to group delivery. Discussing different approaches to group delivery can encourage others to try out new approaches.

9.3 Additional training needs

For any individual working with food it is important to have an up-to-date food hygiene/safety certificate and for those encouraging an increase in physical activity, seeking a qualification to support this would be appropriate, for example Exercise to Music at level 3.

If working with children or vulnerable adults, an up-to-date criminal records check will be required.

For additional skills the facilitator may wish to consider training in specific areas that are going to be beneficial to their ability to help people make lifestyle changes. The need for these additional skills may have been identified through the reflection, peer observation or evaluation process.

Examples include:

- Active listening skills
- Understanding behaviour change
- Motivational interviewing
- Solution focussed practice
- Emotional intelligence
- How to raise awareness of the need to change behaviours
- Presentation skills
- Inclusive teaching
- Cultural awareness
- Conflict resolution.

The value of these different skills have been discussed in previous chapters.

TOP TIP: REFLECTION, PEER OBSERVATION AND EVALUATION SHOULD BE USED TO IDENTIFY ADDITIONAL TRAINING NEEDS

Examples:

Case-study 1:

The group facilitator is new to facilitating groups where the members are of a different ethnicity to those they normally work with. A colleague is observing the group experience and when they feedback they comment on the fact that some of the foods suggested were not appropriate for people of the given cultural background. They also mention that women in the group would find it difficult to increase their physical activity levels unless it was a women's only exercise group.

The group facilitator reflects on the feedback and as part of their action plan looks at the access and availability of cultural awareness training and gains their managers permission to book onto the next course which is available to them.

Case-study 2:

The group facilitator was finding it very difficult to raise the issue of weight management with a group of pregnant women. On the one hand, they knew that excessive gestational weight gain could be harmful to both the mother's and baby's health but on the other hand, they did not want to affect their professional relationship with the mothers. Through reflecting on this feeling they were able to access some e-learning that enabled them to raise the issue of weight management in a sensitive but accurate manner.

In the UK, organizations such as the Royal Society for Public Health (RSPH) offer an excellent range of qualifications, at different levels, for people who are aiming to promote better health. Also, professional organizations offer short courses aimed at both registered staff and assistants. Higher Education Institutes such as universities and colleges may also provide suitable courses that will enhance skills, so it is important to make time to look at the courses that are available, suit one's individual requirements and are accessible. For anyone wishing to combine their practice development with additional academic qualifications, evaluating their practice offers an opportunity to tick both boxes.

TOP TIP: COMBINE PRACTICE, PROFESSIONAL AND ACADEMIC DEVELOPMENT, A CASE-STUDY

The group facilitator identified, as part of their professional development, the need and has undertaken additional training in motivational interviewing.

As part of a Masters course they are undertaking at a local university, they are evaluating the effect of this additional training on the outcomes reported from a weight management group. The research will report on before and after qualitative and quantitative outcomes.

This example could be applied to other training which may have been undertaken, for example the use of emotional intelligence or understanding behaviour change where one could also evaluate before and after outcomes.

There are also bespoke training opportunities for group facilitation skills, which are accredited with the Institute for Leadership and Management (see www.ica-uk.org.uk). Local further education colleges may offer a range of different teaching qualifications, offered at different levels. E-learning is another option. For example, those wanting to develop their communication skills can use an open access training package such as: DIET-COMMS www.nottingham.ac.uk/toolkits/play_13244. This training package is designed to support the development and enhancement of communication skills in dietitians and other healthcare professionals. This can be used by individuals or with peers. Again, it is important to make time to look at what courses are available and which courses are going to best meet individual needs. Discussing different opportunities and courses available with colleagues will help identify most suitable options.

To conclude, personal development in facilitating groups is important irrespective of current level of skills and confidence. Reflection and self-evaluation are easily accessed and non-threatening methods but working with colleagues and having a supportive environment for peer review, observation and discussions helps everyone to develop within the team. Some additional training in specific areas may be identified as being required but again remember to share your learning with colleagues. Finally, do keep a personal development portfolio with records of all reflections, peer observations and certificates of attendance from specific training courses.

References

Askew, S. (2004) Learning about teaching through reflective, collaborative enquiry and observation. *Learning Matters*, Institute of Education, Issue 15.

Blackwell R (1996). Peer observation of teaching and professional development. *Higher Education Quarterly* 50(2): 156–171.

De Stobbeleir KEM, Ashford SJ and Buyens D (2011). Self-regulation of creativity at work: the role of feedback-seeking behaviour in creative performance. *Acad Manage J* 54(4): 811–831.

Driscoll J (2007). *Practising Clinical Supervision: A Reflective Approach for Healthcare Professionals*. Philadelphia, PA: Elsevier.

Gibbs G (1988). *Learning by Doing: A Guide to Teaching and Learning Methods*. Oxford: Further Education Unit Oxford Polytechnic.

Morrison EW (1993). Newcomer information seeking: Exploring types, modes, sources, and outcomes. *Acad Manage J* 36(3): 557–589.

Index

How to Facilitate Lifestyle Change: Applying Group Education in Healthcare, First Edition.
Amanda Avery, Kirsten Whitehead and Vanessa Halliday.
© 2017 John Wiley & Sons, Ltd. Published 2017 by John Wiley & Sons, Ltd.